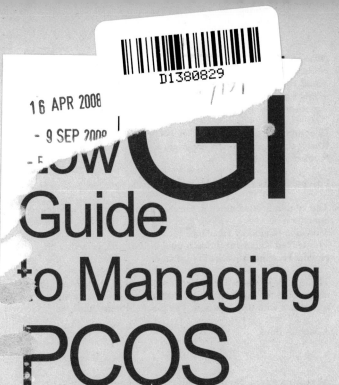

Low GI Guide to Managing PCOS

Dr Jennie Brand-Miller
authority on low GI eating
Prof. Nadir R. Farid, Kate Marsh

Recipes by Alison Roberts and Tracy Rutherford
Consulting Dietician: Elana Hirschowitz

Lose Weight, Boost Fertility and Take
Control with this Easy-to-Follow Diet
and Lifestyle Programme

HODDER

MOBIUS

Copyright © Jennie Brand-Miller, Nadir Farid and Kate Marsh 2004
Recipes on pages 137–185 copyright © Alison Roberts and Tracy Rutherford 2004

First published by Hodder Headline Australia

This edition first published in Great Britain in 2005 by Hodder and Stoughton
A division of Hodder Headline
This United Kingdom edition is published by arrangement with Hodder Headline Australia Pty Limited

The right of Jennie Brand-Miller, Nadir Farid and Kate Marsh to be identified as the Authors of the Work has been asserted by them in accordance with the Copyright, Designs and Patents Act 1988

A Mobius Book

5

A CIP catalogue record for this title is available from the British Library

ISBN 978-0-340-89601-3

Text design and typesetting by Egan-Reid Ltd, Auckland

Printed and bound by Clays Lt

Hodder Headline's policy is to recyclable products and made f
The logging and manufacturin
to the environmental regulatio

Hodder and Stoughton Ltd
A division of Hodder Headlin
338 Euston Road
London NW1 3BH

CONTENTS

CHAPTER 4 PUTTING THE GI TO WORK IN YOUR DAY

CHAPTER 5 RECIPES

ACKNOWLEDGMENTS

Books like this don't happen on their own. Everyone at Hodder Headine Australia deserves a medal for professionalism, but we want to single out Senior Editor, Siobhan Gooley, who gave it everything she had. For the details of coordinating this UK edition we also want to thank Publishing and Production Manager Fiona Hazard and Project Editor Anna Waddington.

Professor Jennie Brand-Miller
I am indebted to Dr Warren Kidson who encouraged and inspired me to write this book. Dr Kidson was one of the first endocrinologists in the world to recognise that women with PCOS were not only insulin resistant but that improving insulin sensitivity was the key to management.

Professor Nadir R. Farid
I am grateful to Ms Elana Hirschowitz, who convinced me how a properly explained low GI diet can work miracles, and Dr Anna Louise Shankland who, despite being a young busy doctor, showed how a low GI diet works like a dream!

Kate Marsh
My inspiration for this book came from talking to hundreds of women who struggle with PCOS and from Dr Warren Kidson who recognised that a low GI diet can make a difference.

INTRODUCTION

Why we wrote this book

Chances are you've picked up this book because you, or your doctor, suspect that you have PCOS—the popular shorthand for polycystic ovarian syndrome—and you want to find out more about it.

No doubt you have plenty of questions and want some simple, straightforward answers. What exactly is PCOS? What are the signs and symptoms? How is the diagnosis confirmed? What causes it? Why *you*? And most importantly, what can you do about it? These are the type of questions we often get asked as professionals working daily with women with PCOS.

We wrote this book to try and give you some answers, and to give you the practical tools you need to help improve the underlying cause of PCOS: insulin resistance— a condition in which the body resists the actions of the hormone insulin.

What's more, we'll show you *how* you can improve your insulin sensitivity, step by step, with a delicious low GI diet that's so effective, you'll want to stick to it for life. Not only will you lose weight in the first few months, you'll eat till you're satisfied and you'll never feel hungry. And none of your favourite foods are excluded entirely. Once you've lost weight, we do what other diet books don't—we give you a long-term eating plan to ensure you keep that weight off for life. And we explain how the GI fits in with other health messages about different types of fat and protein, showing you how easy it is to expand your healthy eating choices.

Diet won't be the only thing you change, of course. Exercise and medication are also important tools, but without key dietary changes, you'll be doing it the hard way. So, congratulate yourself, you've picked the right book to start managing your PCOS. As you read on you'll discover lots of real life stories showing exactly how exercise, healthy low GI eating and the right medication can balance hormones, reduce insulin resistance, help beat the symptoms of PCOS and, best of all, enable you to take charge.

About us

Jennie has been researching all aspects of carbohydrates—diet and diabetes, the glycaemic index of foods, insulin resistance—for over 20 years. Her authoritative, internationally bestselling series on the glycaemic index, *The New Glucose Revolution* (which also incorporates The Low GI Guides) which she wrote with Kaye Foster-Powell and Professor Stephen Colagiuri has sold over three million copies worldwide, and been translated into 14 languages. The scientific evidence that the GI is important for health is now beyond dispute and Jennie's ongoing research includes the role of a low GI diet in relieving the symptoms of PCOS.

Nadir is an internationally recognised investigative and clinical endocrinologist. His groundbreaking work has led to a greater understanding of PCOS and improved medical treatment for women with PCOS. More recently he has been independently researching the role of low GI diets in the treatment of PCOS.

Kate has met and helped hundreds of women with PCOS through her work in private practice since 1997. She is currently undertaking her PhD at the University of

Sydney looking at the benefits of a low GI diet in the management of insulin resistance in women with PCOS.

What's so different about *The New Glucose Revolution*?

The New Glucose Revolution is a lifelong eating plan, not a calorie-restrictive diet. It's a groundbreaking way of eating based on what is known as the glycaemic index (GI), which is the scientifically proven way of describing how carbohydrates in individual foods affect blood glucose levels. What you need to understand about the GI is that:

- Foods containing carbohydrates that break down quickly during digestion, releasing glucose quickly into the bloodstream, have a high GI.

- Foods that contain carbohydrates that break down slowly, releasing glucose into the bloodstream gradually, have a low GI.

Low GI foods are our key to unlocking the benefits of *The New Glucose Revolution* and achieving weight loss and blood glucose control. In turn, these will lead to more effective management of your PCOS symptoms. If you make the change and base your diet around healthy low GI foods you will achieve lower insulin levels, making it easier for your body to burn fat and less likely that fat will be stored. Eating plenty of healthy low GI foods will also:

- help lower your blood fats

- make you feel 'full' and thus reduce appetite

- reduce your risk of developing diabetes

- improve your overall health

These aren't claims. These are facts that have been confirmed in numerous worldwide scientific studies.

In *The Low GI Guide to Managing PCOS* we show you how easy it is to include more of the right sort of low GI carbohydrates in your diet everyday and in every meal; which common foods have a low GI; and how you can make the GI work for you throughout the day with:

- practical hints for changing your eating habits

- quick and easy, healthy, low GI, low kilojoule recipes, meal ideas and snacks

You are not alone

If you have PCOS you are not alone. Elements of PCOS are thought to affect one in four women in developed nations. The severe form affects one in twenty. At the root of PCOS is insulin resistance. In chapter one, we explain exactly what insulin resistance is. We also show you that there's plenty you can do about it, starting with diet and exercise.

INSULIN RESISTANCE

Insulin resistance is at the root of PCOS. We now know that more than half the population is insulin resistant—men and women, young and old. Insulin resistance is a chameleon that shows itself in many ways, differing from one person to another and between men and women. At one extreme, an individual may have only mildly abnormal blood tests. At the other, she (or he) may have a severe condition such as diabetes that impacts negatively on health, quality of life and life expectancy. For more information see www.diagnosemefirst.com.

And remember: a diet that is good for anyone who has PCOS, is a diet that's good for everybody, every day, every meal.

The signs of PCOS range from subtle symptoms, such as faint facial hair, to a 'full house' syndrome—lack of periods, infertility, heavy body-hair growth, obstinate body fat, diabetes and cardiovascular disease.

The symptoms of PCOS can occur at any age. Insulin resistance rises naturally at puberty, so PCOS can be seen in girls as young as 10 or 12 years old. What's more, it does not suddenly disappear when the ovaries retire at menopause. Management of insulin resistance should continue beyond menopause as a supplement to other health-enhancing lifestyle measures.

It's vital to diagnose and treat women and girls as early as possible in order to prevent their PCOS progressing to the 'full house' syndrome. The outdated view that early signs are 'clinically insignificant' and not worthy of proper management is simply not true. In fact, the sooner you (and your doctor) act, the better. As well as advice on medical management, diet and exercise, we also offer you tips on overcoming the stress and sleep problems that come hand in hand with PCOS. This is a total lifestyle plan for helping you manage your PCOS. It's your choice to adopt a programme that ensures your present and future health. We have written this book to help you make that choice.

Knowledge is definitely power when it comes to your health. So, first up, we answer those pressing questions women ask about PCOS, its causes and medical management. In Chapter 2 we get down to detail on understanding the glycaemic index, or GI for short, and the diet revolution we have been part of for over 20 years. A diet revolution that is now taking the whole world by storm. For the practical know-how to put it all into practice day by day, turn to Chapter 3 and check out the expert advice from a dietitian with more experience in managing PCOS than just about anyone else around. And finally we fill you up with delicious low GI recipes specially devised by Alison Roberts and Tracy Rutherford that you will enjoy preparing time and again as you reap the benefits of healthy low GI eating.

We believe understanding is very important if you are going to take charge and manage your PCOS, so we have included a glossary of technical terms at the back of the book as a quick reference. In the further reading section you will also find a list of organisations that will provide you with support and put you in contact with other women with PCOS, plus lots of websites and references you can follow up if you want to find out more.

CHAPTER 1

UNDERSTANDING PCOS

How can I tell if I have PCOS?
A little history
PCOS is more common than you'd expect
Doctors have to suspect it to diagnose it
The insulin resistance link
What exactly is insulin resistance?
How does excess insulin cause PCOS?
How insulin causes excess body fat
Can you inherit insulin resistance?
Why is insulin resistance so common?
PCOS is a risk factor for further medical complications
Signs of the insulin resistance syndrome
Effective medical management of PCOS
A much-wanted pregnancy
Skin and hair
The longer term

How can I tell if I have PCOS?

Only a doctor can diagnose PCOS. But here's a list of the subtle symptoms of PCOS—not all of which need be present:

- delayed (or early) puberty

- irregular or no periods

- acne

- excess body or facial hair

- unexplained fatigue

- sugar craving

- hypoglycemia: (low blood glucose) after meals. The most common symptoms are light-headedness, sweating, sudden fatigue and butterflies in the tummy

- excess weight around the waistline

- infertility

- mood swings

- hot flushes (heat intolerance and excess sweating) in young women

- sleep disorders: such as sleep apnoea

- recurrent spontaneous miscarriages

- inappropriate lactation

- drop in blood pressure on standing up suddenly or with exercise

- acanthosis nigricans: rough, dark skin in the neck folds and armpits; a mark of severe insulin resistance from any cause

If you have one or more of these signs or symptoms, you should make an appointment with your doctor. They may refer you to an endocrinologist who specialises in PCOS.

A little history

Although polycystic ovaries were first described in France way back in 1844, it was two New York gynaecologists, Irving F. Stein and Michael L. Leventhal, who diagnosed women with what we now consider to be severe PCOS and coined the term in 1935. The women that they described suffered from amenorrhea (no periods), severe hirsutism (unwanted hair) and polycystic ovaries (large ovaries with multiple cysts).

PCOS is more common than you'd expect

Up to one in four women in industrialised countries have certain features of PCOS and the vast majority of them do not even suspect it. PCOS should be suspected in anyone with excess weight around the waist, excessive hair in the wrong places, acne, irregular periods, no periods or problems getting pregnant. Young women who require insulin to control their diabetes are also at risk of developing PCOS.

Symptoms of PCOS usually first appear around menarche (the first period), but can occur anytime during a woman's reproductive life. Subtle symptoms such as hot flushes (long before menopause), otherwise unexplained weight gain, mood swings, hirsutism and 'hypoglycemia' (low blood glucose) after meals may be suggestive of PCOS. Despite its name, PCOS involves the whole body and not just the ovaries. This is why it is so important to identify girls who are at risk *before* they reach puberty. If PCOS can be treated early, there are lifelong health benefits.

THE NORMAL FEMALE CYCLE

To understand PCOS you need to understand the normal menstrual cycle.

The hypothalamus in the brain signals the pituitary gland to secrete FSH (follicle-stimulating hormone) and LH (luteinising hormone). In the first half of the cycle, these pulses are infrequent and FSH is secreted preferentially, allowing a crop of follicles to grow inside the ovaries. This phase is therefore called the 'follicular' phase. The follicles secrete estrogen and acquire receptors for LH. As estrogen levels rise, the hypothalamus pulses more and more frequently. Estrogen stimulates the growth of the breasts and of the lining of the uterus. Most of the follicles degenerate in the next few days and only one is mysteriously selected. This dominant follicle (the 'egg') matures over the next few days and just before ovulation—when the dominant follicle is expelled from the ovary—estrogen levels peak.

After ovulation, the dominant ruptured follicle becomes the corpus luteum. This little body secretes progesterone, the hormone that promotes the growth of blood vessels of the uterine lining in preparation of the implanting of a fertilised egg. This phase is called the luteal phase. If the egg is not fertilised, estrogen and progesterone levels fall, and the uterine lining is shed and menstruation occurs. At the time of puberty when girls have reached a critical muscle-to-fat ratio, the hypothalamus gives the GO signal for the start of menstruation. Excessive weight loss, exercise or stress can negate that signal.

At the peak years of reproductive life most women have a regular 28-day cycle, plus or minus 2–3 days. The first day of the menstrual period is day 1. Ovulation usually occurs on day 14 to 15, but can occur anywhere from day 9 to 17 due to variability in the length of the follicular phase of the cycle. Around menarche and menopause, the cycles are irregular and often not associated with ovulation.

The ovary is a sensitive beacon for insulin resistance and thus allows early recognition of a metabolic problem. Having PCOS increases the likelihood that further medical problems will develop over time. These include: type 2 diabetes, heart disease, hypertension, fatty liver and cancer of the uterus. We also know that serious sleep disorders and depression are much more common in women with PCOS. Alarmingly, women with PCOS who do get pregnant stand a 40 per cent chance of spontaneous miscarriage in the first three months of pregnancy. There is also an increased risk of gestational diabetes, multiple pregnancies and in later pregnancy, pre-eclampsia (a serious complication of late pregnancy which requires immediate medical attention). When a thorough medical check was carried out after delivery, a high percentage of women with gestational diabetes were found to have PCOS. Although direct evidence is not available, some doctors even suspect that PCOS will turn out to be a risk factor for Alzheimer's disease. Women with PCOS are also at an increased risk for autoimmune thyroid disease resulting in underactive or overactive thyroid.

Given the fact that it afflicts up to 25 per cent of women of reproductive age, PCOS should be considered a health hazard for all women. Indeed, one wonders if it should be called a disease at all—PCOS is more than just a personal problem, because it affects so many women. It needs to be seen as a public health issue that deserves community support.

Doctors have to suspect it to diagnose it

The sooner you have a definite diagnosis of PCOS the better. That's because intervention and treatment will be more effective if 'the full house' of symptoms has not yet set in. This requires a high level of suspicion on the part of your doctor. Here are the test results that should alert your doctor:

- A blood test showing that key hormones are abnormally high or low: testosterone that is too high, high levels of luteinising hormone (LH) while follicle-stimulating hormone (FSH) levels are normal. Most women seen today have normal FSH and LH levels.

- An ultrasound examination showing 'bulky' ovaries with 10 or more peripheral cysts. In thin women, ultrasound through the abdominal wall will allow good views of uterus and ovaries but for those who are overweight, internal ultrasound examination is often necessary.

It is important to stress that the symptoms, blood test results and ultrasound findings need to be interpreted by a medical practitioner with experience in PCOS. Some women do not show the 'classic' signs at all. Indeed, some women with classic PCOS may ovulate frequently and perhaps regularly.

Some doctors make a distinction between polycystic ovarian *syndrome* (PCOS) and polycystic ovarian *disease* (PCOD). You may have heard both terms used. Both PCOS and PCOD are underpinned by the same metabolic problem—insulin resistance. They have to be treated in much the same way. For simplicity, throughout this book, we use the term PCOS to refer to both.

The insulin resistance link

Insulin resistance is a condition in which the body 'resists' the normal actions of the hormone insulin, that is, the body's response to insulin is defective. To overcome this resistance, the body secretes more insulin than normal. The vast majority of women with PCOS have severe insulin

My Mum recommended that I see the doctor because I was trying to get pregnant (I had been married for nine months) but wasn't having much success. My periods were regular but they were longer than usual. I also had dark hairs growing up the naval line as well as on the inside of my upper thighs below the bikini-line. Because the hair growth was of recent onset, he immediately suspected PCOS, and sent me off for an ultrasound later the same afternoon. The ultrasound confirmed that both ovaries, but more so the right, were enlarged and contained multiple cysts.

I had some blood tests too which were suggestive of PCOS. He prescribed a healthy low GI diet, exercise and metformin tablets. A few weeks later I went on a dream holiday to the Caribbean for two weeks, and on my return I was delighted to discover that I was pregnant! I have continued with the healthy low GI diet and exercise programme and I plan to stick to it for life.

Louise, 27

resistance and may have high insulin levels. Simple measurements relating fasting blood sugar to insulin have not been found to be helpful in diagnosing insulin resistance, as has been suggested until quite recently.

Being overweight or obese increases the degree of insulin resistance, but you can be very lean and still have PCOS (and be insulin resistant). You could also have PCOS as a result of an unusual inherited or acquired disease of the adrenal glands—it's pretty rare, but it should be considered by your doctor as part of the medical investigations as it requires specific treatment for the primary underlying condition. Women with PCOS also secrete more than normal amounts of sex steroids from both the ovaries and the adrenal glands.

What exactly is insulin resistance?

Whenever we eat, whatever the nature of the food, glucose and insulin levels in the blood rise and fall over the next couple of hours. Both carbohydrates and proteins in our food stimulate the secretion of insulin—it is essential for life. Insulin drives the transport of glucose (from digested carbohydrate) and amino acids (the building blocks of protein) into our cells, as well as the storage of glucose in the liver and our muscles.

Insulin can also suppress the use of fat as a source of fuel and the capacity of the liver to make new glucose molecules—neither of which are needed during the first hour or two after a meal. Think of insulin as a facilitator of 'energy storage'.

Beyond these roles in metabolism, insulin is important for growth before and after birth, and it's absolutely essential for the optimal functioning of many other hormones and enzymes. We are also beginning to learn about the role insulin plays in brain function, and thus behaviour. Insulin has functions in our bodies besides carbohydrate metabolism, so it comes as no surprise that insulin resistance is associated with infiltration of muscle (including heart muscle), and in severe cases the liver, with fats and with abnormalities in blood lipids and other body chemistries.

Like a lock and key mechanism, most body cells have special 'receptors' for insulin. Once the lock is engaged—insulin attaches itself to the receptor—the gates open, allowing glucose to flow into the cell. The higher the concentration of insulin receptors, the more insulin sensitive you are.

If the number of insulin receptors is lower than normal or they are compromised in some way, then the cells are said to be 'insulin resistant'. The pancreas, the organ that secretes insulin, responds to this situation by secreting more insulin in an effort to overcome the block and achieve normal transport of glucose. One of the hallmarks of insulin resistance is therefore an inappropriately high level of insulin in the blood, both before and after meals.

Unfortunately, in many people, the pancreas has a limited capacity to secrete large amounts of insulin. It is only a matter of time before the cells burn out and they can't supply enough insulin to meet demand and the person develops pre-diabetes or the full-blown diabetic state. On the other hand reducing insulin resistance can delay those states.

How does excess insulin cause PCOS?

Great progress is being made in understanding the links between excess insulin and PCOS. Insulin stimulates the growth and multiplication of cells in the ovary, in particular those that make up the bulk of the ovary in which the eggs are embedded. Insulin resistance leads to a vicious cycle of hormonal imbalances which create the symptoms of PCOS.

The receptors for insulin in the ovary are different from those in other tissues, in that when blood insulin levels are high, the ovary does not turn down insulin receptor numbers or reduce their activity. Therefore, the action of insulin continues unabated in ovarian tissues. The cells grow and multiply, as well as increasing their metabolic activity. The result is excessive production of both male (testosterone) as well as female (estrogen) sex hormones. When the body is functioning healthily, men and women produce both sorts of hormones although in vastly different proportions.

> Insulin resistance leads to a vicious cycle of hormonal imbalances which create the symptoms of PCOS.

Normally, the ovary makes testosterone and then converts it to estrogen. However, excessive stimulation of the ovary overwhelms its capacity to fully undertake this conversion, with the result that excess testosterone spills over into the blood. The uncharacteristically high testosterone levels in the blood then bring about 'male' characteristics in women, such as hirsutism and weight gain. Most women with PCOS also produce excessive male hormones from the adrenal glands.

Excess insulin and sex hormones also work together to stimulate one of the areas in the brain called the hypothalamus, making it more sensitive. It 'pulses' more frequently than normal, inducing the gland underneath—called the pituitary—to secrete more luteinising hormone (LH for short). LH stimulates the ovary's hormone production even more—and a vicious cycle is up and running. Breaking that cycle is the key to managing PCOS successfully.

Excess insulin has even more consequences. It stimulates the conversion of weak male and female hormones to the more potent forms—estrogen and testosterone. And, finally, it reduces the level of the protein that binds testosterone in the blood. In this way, the active form of the hormone is made 'more available' to the tissues.

Testosterone is called an anabolic hormone because it is involved in building up new tissues, especially muscles. This muscle-building potential is the main reason men have more muscle mass than women. It's also why unscrupulous athletes use it to enhance their performance. In women with PCOS, however, excess testosterone and other male hormones contribute to excessive weight gain and 'masculinisation'.

It is this complicated interplay between insulin resistance, ovarian hormones and increased pituitary stimulation of the ovaries that accounts for all the signs and hormonal features of PCOS.

How insulin causes excess body fat

Fat cells and their precursor cells in different parts of the human body are not all the same. Those around the midriff and inside the tummy are particularly sensitive to the effects of insulin compared with those in the rest of the body.

One of insulin's most powerful actions is to inhibit the release of fat from fat stores, making it difficult to call on abdominal fat as a source of fuel. In this way, midriff fat gradually accumulates around the waist, a sign that is typical of women and girls with PCOS. In fact, it is one of the most obvious and typical signs of insulin resistance in both women and men.

Can you inherit insulin resistance?

We know that insulin resistance is more common in some groups of people than others. For example, Asian people have been found to be more insulin resistant than people

'PCOS' IN MEN

Some studies have shown the 'trait' associated with PCOS in women members of a family also appeared to be passed on to some of the men in that family. Men are as liable to insulin resistance as women, but not having ovaries, the signs of the disease are different. Frontal baldness and, to a lesser measure, excessive body-hair growth, was once thought to indicate insulin resistance in male relatives; more recent studies have demonstrated that these factors are not reliable indicators of 'PCOS in men'. Rather it manifests itself as central obesity, carbohydrate craving, fatigue, sleep disorders, dyslipidaemia (see Glossary on page 203) and fatty liver. Also, raised serum androstenedione has been found to be a tell-tale sign for affected male relatives.

of Caucasian origin. And American Indians, Australian Aborigines and Pacific Islanders are more insulin resistant than most.

Not surprisingly, PCOS also runs in families and often there is a family history of type 2 diabetes too. Modern genetic analyses point the finger at several genes which suggest a predisposition to PCOS, but one of them in isolation is not sufficient to cause the disease. Many of the genes identified are involved in the action of insulin and in the production or metabolism of the sex hormones. So, to some extent you can blame your genes—and your parents!

Environmental factors and lack of physical exercise are also important. We know that weight gain can trigger insulin resistance and PCOS as can steroid medication. Apparently stress can induce changes in many cells in the body that initiate and propagate insulin resistance; in addition stress speeds up genetic changes associated with aging, also known to be a factor in insulin resistance. We are less sure about the links between PCOS and the use of contraceptives.

If you were born small—with a birth weight under 2.5 kg (5½ pounds)—you are more likely to be insulin resistant. Baby girls with low birth weight who then put on weight quickly within the first year or two of life, are especially likely to develop PCOS at the time of their first period. Indeed, there is evidence that babies of PCOS mothers exposed to high levels of insulin and androgen while in the womb exhibit evidence of insulin resistance before puberty.

> PCOS also runs in families and often there is a family history of type 2 diabetes.

Why is insulin resistance so common?

Many of the women with PCOS that we meet wonder why something so seemingly undesirable would be so common and have a genetic basis. One popular theory that endeavours to explain the prevalence of insulin resistance is called the 'thrifty genotype' hypothesis. According to this theory, our ancestors endured cycles of food scarcity and food abundance. Those individuals with a degree of insulin resistance had an advantage because their high insulin levels suppressed the use of fat as a fuel source, leading to greater body fat accumulation during periods of abundance. Then, when food was scarce, they could draw on those fat reserves. This survival advantage meant the genes for insulin resistance (i.e. the 'thrifty' genes) spread throughout human populations.

An alternative theory, called the 'carnivore connection' is gaining ground. According to this theory, genes for insulin resistance were particularly advantageous during the Ice Ages that characterised the last two million years of human evolution. When the planet was colder and drier, and plant growth was limited, human diets are thought to have become increasingly carnivorous—dependent on the large herds of animals that thrived on the steppes of Europe and the grasslands of Africa. Such diets are low in carbohydrates. Hence a metabolism that spared blood glucose for essential purposes, redirecting it away from muscles, would have had survival and reproductive advantages. The large human brain and the foetus are both exclusively dependent on glucose as a source of fuel—they cannot use fat. On this diet, the genes for insulin resistance may have become more and more common.

Whatever the reason—food scarcity in general, or just carbohydrates in short supply—it's clear that the genes for insulin resistance are no longer an advantage. In developed nations, food is too plentiful and our lifestyles too sedentary and more stressful, and those previously advantageous metabolic attributes have come to prey upon our health. We have made our lifestyles just too easy for our own good.

I was referred to the endocrinologist because I often had dizzy turns and my GP found one of two fasting blood glucose levels were a bit low. I went with my mum, Diane, because I am rather shy and hate seeing doctors. The endocrinologist asked lots of questions and made me realise that I often felt light-headed, faint and sweaty about two hours after some meals. He also pointed out that I was slightly underweight and had mild excess body-hair growth. Although my blood pressure was normal, it showed a significant drop when he measured it as I was standing and that's when I felt faint. He found that I was insulin resistant and arranged for an ultrasound that day which showed that I had large polycystic ovaries. That's when he prescribed metformin plus a healthy low GI diet with lots of vegetables and regular aerobic exercise (which I hate!).

Ruth, 18

My daughter Ruth was having dizzy spells, so I went to the doctor with her and that's when I learned all about insulin resistance and the fact that it runs in families. So I booked myself in to see the endocrinologist straightaway. I am post-menopausal and a survivor of large bowel cancer. I am also a bit overweight (the endocrinologist called it 'centrally obese'). I have high blood pressure too. After examining me and sending me off for all sorts of tests, the doctor realised that I had all the signs of the metabolic syndrome including high cholesterol, low 'good cholesterol' and high triglycerides, and high blood glucose two hours after a glucose drink. My heart tracing showed evidence of an old heart attack. He put me on metformin, a healthy low GI diet, blood pressure tablets and medications to lower my blood fats. And, of course, an exercise programme.

Diane, 48

Insulin resistance is now regarded as the underlying basis for all the diseases of affluence: obesity, pre-diabetes, type 2 diabetes, abnormal cholesterol levels, high blood pressure, coronary artery disease, fatty liver, pre-eclampsia and PCOS. Who gets them? Disease is determined by your gender, diet, lifestyle and how overweight you are—together with all those other genes you inherited from your mum and dad.

PCOS is a risk factor for further medical complications

Reducing your insulin resistance is vital, not only for tackling the symptoms of PCOS but also to minimise the complications that often follow on from insulin resistance. We want to emphasise that some of these risks are worst-case scenarios and can be prevented by the type of treatment and sensible lifestyle changes recommended in this book.

- the insulin resistance/metabolic syndrome

- type 2 diabetes

- thyroid disease leading to underactive and overactive thyroid

- coronary artery disease

- stroke

- early miscarriages

- multiple pregnancies

- pre-eclampsia

- uterine cancer

- depression

- Alzheimer's disease

Signs of the insulin resistance syndrome

Doctors can pinpoint the metabolic characteristics of anyone with *severe* insulin resistance. These days it's called the 'metabolic syndrome' but it also goes by the name of 'Syndrome X'. If you have this syndrome, you won't necessarily show every characteristic listed below, but you will have at least two or three of them:

- a large waist circumference (also known as central obesity)

- high blood glucose (in the fasting state before breakfast or after meals)

- high blood pressure

- high blood triglyceride ('trigs')

- high levels of small, dense cholesterol

- low levels of HDL (the good cholesterol)

- fatty liver (non-alcoholic steatohepatitis or NASH)

- PCOS

Left undiagnosed and untreated, a person with the metabolic syndrome will often go on to develop other more serious medical problems (see list on page 21).

Effective medical management of PCOS

The vast majority of women with PCOS are profoundly insulin resistant even if they are not overweight. Managing their PCOS requires an integrated programme of lifestyle change and medication to achieve the treatment goals: weight loss if necessary, normalising blood hormone levels, control of acne, resumption of ovulation and regular periods.

METFORMIN

Metformin has been around for a long time. In fact it has been used to treat people with type 2 diabetes for over 50 years. It has recently gained greater respect because we now know that it also helps to prevent the long-term complications of diabetes, such as eye and coronary artery diseases.

Metformin works by reducing glucose production by the liver and increasing the uptake of glucose by the body (i.e. it increases insulin sensitivity). This is why it is so useful in treating women with PCOS. In fact, even before a woman with PCOS has achieved any significant weight loss, metformin can be effective in improving her other symptoms.

There are some side effects, however, including a metallic taste in the mouth, nausea, excess gas and soft stools that may graduate to diarrhoea. For most people, these are mild and disappear within a few weeks. However, to keep any possible side effects and discomfort to a mimimum, doctors usually introduce metformin gradually over a period of three to four weeks starting with a 500 milligram tablet after dinner for ten days. If this causes no major problems then another 500 milligram tablet is introduced after breakfast and in another ten days another tablet is taken after lunch. Some women prefer to take their medication only twice a day and use 850 milligram tablets twice a day. The optimal dose is around 1500–1700 milligrams per day.

Metformin may interfere with the absorption of vitamin B12. Hence it is important to have regular blood tests to measure blood levels of B12 and liver function tests. Taking calcium can apparently protect against the drop in serum B12 related to metformin. If you have kidney or liver failure or serious circulatory problems, you should not take metformin at all.

It should be noted that in most countries, no drug other than the contraceptive pill is licensed for the treatment of PCOS. Even metformin is not yet approved for this purpose.

The cornerstone of managing PCOS is lifestyle modification with a healthy low GI diet and exercise. These changes need to be initiated right from the start, even before the use of insulin-sensitising drugs.

It is also important to keep in mind that your treatment should be tailored to deal with your symptoms and, to some extent, your priorities. That might be regular periods, a much-wanted pregnancy or simply a reduction in body hair.

Until recently, the most popular medical approach of treating PCOS was to 'suppress ovarian function and replace estrogen' with an oral contraceptive pill (such as Dianette). While this is effective, it does nothing to address the basic problem of insulin resistance, the underlying cause of PCOS. Moreover, because estrogen is one of the two components in the pill, long-term use carries the same risk as that for estrogen alone, including the risk of breast cancer.

In recent years, and with a better understanding of the metabolic basis of PCOS, the emphasis has shifted. Many doctors now direct their efforts to managing insulin resistance in PCOS with an integrated programme of low GI diet, regular aerobic exercises and insulin-sensitising drugs such as metformin.

Taking metformin in a final optimal dose of 500 milligrams three times a day with meals generally produces a very satisfying result including weight loss, normalisation of hormonal levels (testosterone, LH and insulin), resumption of regular periods, ovulation and pregnancy. But the key to success is early diagnosis and treatment combined with a low GI diet and exercise.

The uterine wall in women with PCOS who fall pregnant does not produce a substance (glycodelin) that suppresses the immune system so the early foetus is not rejected. Metformin promotes the production of glycodelin, which

I am a volunteer worker, and I had already been to a couple of clinics in the last few years to see what could be done about my weight gain, lack of periods (amenorrhea) and high blood pressure. Although someone mentioned PCOS at some stage, it wasn't followed up. I was really concerned about my health and especially my weight (I weighed 97 kilograms (214 pounds) and am only 155 centimetres (5ft 1″)) and my GP sent me to see an endocrinologist. They did lots of tests and found that I was mildly hypertensive and had rough skin at the root of the neck and particularly under my armpits (acanthosis nigricans). I also had stretch marks on my tummy and upper thighs. They found that I had an LH level of 46 and FSH of 3.6 mU/L, serum testosterone three times the upper limit of the normal range. My fasting insulin was also high, when related to blood glucose drawn at the same time. Various procedures including an internal ultrasound, laproscopy and biopsy confirmed that I had really severe PCOS. I was prescribed metformin and blood pressure medication and instructed on how to follow a healthy low GI diet. I was also told that I must do some aerobic exercise every day and I opted for swimming. My symptoms improved slightly but I was intolerant to more than 500 milligrams of metformin a day so they changed me over to a newer 'heavy duty' insulin sensitising drug called Roziglitazone™ (Avandia©). Regular monitoring is essential with this and I have to have monthly liver function testing and use barrier contraception as the impact of this medication on the foetus is unknown. Over the next six weeks the dosage of Avandia© was built up to maximum and in three months I had been able to lose 8 kilograms (17½ pounds) and my acanthosis nigricans improved markedly. Amazingly, a month later, I had my first period in 12 years!

Helen, 29

may explain its protective influence against early foetal loss. For women who fall pregnant, some doctors advocate that metformin be continued through the first 12 weeks (or more) of pregnancy to prevent the otherwise high likelihood of miscarriage. Other doctors suggest that metformin is stopped once the woman is pregnant. At present there is no control research to favour either recommendation.

Although metformin is a category B drug (safety in pregnancy not demonstrated) there is no evidence to date that it harms the foetus, or the child's development after birth.

In due course, newer insulin sensitisers that are more potent than metformin may become useful in the management of PCOS, either alone or in combination with metformin.

A newer class of drugs called thiazolidinediones (e.g. Roziglitazone™ and Pioglitazone™) is being used successfully in the treatment of type 2 diabetes and the metabolic syndrome. These drugs work by sensitising tissues to insulin and may be used in combination with metformin in women with PCOS. Thiazolidinediones should not, however, be used in those who wish to become pregnant.

Combinations of metformin and drugs that block the effect of testosterone on the body (e.g. spiranolactone or finasteride) have also been used in women with severe hirsutism. But, again, these drugs must be avoided for women wanting to fall pregnant.

Drug treatment is also available for the small percentage of women who fail to lose significant amounts of weight, despite their best efforts.

A much-wanted pregnancy

This book is primarily concerned with helping you to manage your PCOS symptoms on a daily basis. Unfortunately, there is not enough space here to have an in-depth look at assisted ovulation and pregnancy in women with PCOS. The measures recommended in this book: a low GI diet, regular exercise and metformin treatment will maximise the likelihood of regular ovulation, and eventually pregnancy. If ovulation is not achieved in four to six months of metformin treatment, other medical intervention should be considered, such as the addition of clomiphene. Indeed, an argument may be made to start clomiphene shortly after metformin in women whose primary concern is pregnancy. The combination works better than either drug alone. Many IVF programmes pre-treat women—even those *without* PCOS—with metformin because it increases the chances of successful embryo implantation.

I consulted my family doctor because I just couldn't get pregnant despite being off the pill for over nine months. I certainly wasn't overweight, although I was a bit tubbier around the tummy than I liked and my periods had been pretty irregular for the last six months. My doctor suspected PCOS and sent me off to have an ultrasound. That showed that both my ovaries were enlarged and had multiple cysts. He prescribed metformin, gave me a programme of aerobic exercises and referred me to a dietitian to learn all about healthy low GI eating. I found the diet really easy to follow and at the same time built up the dose of metformin he had prescribed to a full dose with every meal. It seems amazing now, but just two months after I started this programme I noticed that my tummy was flattening out. Best of all my periods were now regular and I was ovulating. The next month I missed my period. I was pregnant!

Claire, 26

Because even normal pregnancy is an insulin-resistant state, when women with PCOS become pregnant it is all the more reason that they continue to eat a low GI diet, although the calories should be increased to meet the extra needs of the pregnancy. Low GI eating contributes to an enjoyable pregnancy for the mother and a lively, decent-sized baby!

Skin and hair

Acne and an oily complexion, usually appearing around the time of puberty, may be the very first signs of PCOS. Hard-to-treat acne and acne which appears later in life can also signal the possibility of PCOS. Acne associated with PCOS will respond to metformin, although in some cases the addition of antibiotics or androgen blockers may be necessary.

With treatment, excessive facial and body-hair growth will slow down. Hair will become finer as blood levels of the male sex hormones fall. The slow nature of hair growth, however, means that the benefits of any treatment will involve a wait of five to six months. In addition, many women with PCOS are still not satisfied with the level of excess body-hair growth despite metformin treatment and their quality of life is affected. In these cases, testosterone blockers or drugs that influence testosterone metabolism (e.g. flutamide) should be added. Recent studies show that it can be used at a fraction of the traditional dose. Unfortunately, this medication is not without side effects, and liver function tests must be carried out periodically and the drug discontinued if pregnancy is contemplated.

The contraceptive pill is effective in reducing excessive body hair too but using it over a long-term period has been questioned. The water pill, spiranolactone, is less effective, although it has been used for many years at high doses for this purpose.

It may be necessary to supplement the medical treatment of excess facial and body hair with those tried and true traditional methods for hair removal such as depilatory creams, electrolysis, flashlamps, intense pulsed light and laser hair removal. Electrolysis and laser therapy, in particular, often lead to a dramatic improvement in quality of life. The cream 'Vaniqua' when used alongside traditional methods has been found to be effective by most users.

Unfortunately there are many products and procedures, including those for 'permanent hair removal' that do not stand up to the claims of the manufacturers. An excellent guide to appropriate products is: www.hairfacts.com.

The longer term

The longer your insulin resistance remains untreated the more likely you are to develop the metabolic syndrome, type 2 diabetes or cardiovascular disease. Once treatment commences many doctors believe that it is important for women with PCOS to continue medical management longer term and certainly beyond menopause. Lifestyle modification, including a healthy low GI diet, exercise and possibly pharmacological treatment might therefore be lifelong. That makes it all the more critical that the diet and lifestyle you adopt is one you can stick to long term. Anything else will result in the 'rhythm method of girth control'—cycles of weight loss and weight gain that could do more harm than good, not just to your health but to your sense of self-esteem.

This section of the book should have answered all your pressing questions about the causes of PCOS and its medical management. Now it's time to talk in detail about dietary management. In the next chapter we tell you all about the GI, the diet revolution that is taking the whole world by storm.

Summing up

Let's highlight the main points to take home from this chapter.

- Insulin resistance has reached epidemic proportions.

- In women of reproductive age, PCOS is a common manifestation of insulin resistance.

- If not diagnosed early PCOS can progress to a severe form placing women at risk of many serious medical conditions.

- A high index of suspicion for an early diagnosis and effective management is essential.

- As PCOS is a manifestation of insulin resistance, attention to lifestyle must continue past the menopause.

CHAPTER 2

ALL ABOUT CARBOHYDRATES AND THE GI OF FOODS

In this chapter we'll explain the whys and wherefores of making the change to a healthy diet that includes low GI carbohydrates and how this will help you beat the symptoms of PCOS. Women with PCOS or diabetes have often told us that understanding the science behind the insulin connection made it logical and easy to make the change to a healthy low GI diet.

As we showed in the previous chapter, insulin resistance is at the root of PCOS. But, you may well ask, what does this actually do to you? Well, it basically means that your body has a hard time bringing blood glucose levels down after you've eaten—no matter whether it's breakfast, lunch or dinner or just an in-between snack.

This is where what we call *The New Glucose Revolution* comes in. It's a revolution so far-reaching that it will change the way you eat, the way you cook—even the way you think about food. We're talking about the glycaemic index, or the GI as we call it, the scientifically proven way of describing how carbohydrates in individual foods actually affect our blood glucose levels.

The fact is, the GI, which started out as a dietary tool to help people with diabetes choose the right foods to control blood glucose, has become the way of eating that everyone's talking about today—and one of few nutritional programmes with sound scientific research to support it.

Back to basics

The New Glucose Revolution and Low GI Guides make a key contribution to helping you beat PCOS symptoms because it focuses on carbohydrates—their quantity *and* quality, and their overall effect on your blood glucose. Controlling your blood glucose levels is the first step to increasing your insulin sensitivity.

With so much coverage of carbohydrates currently in the media, it's easy to get confused between low carb and high carb diets. Carbohydrates are nature's primary fuel, and a very important food for health and energy.

In our series, *The New Glucose Revolution* and Low GI Guides, we focus not just on carbohydrate quantity—though it is important as you will see later in this chapter—but also on carbohydrate *quality* or, more specifically, the nature of the carbohydrate and its overall effect on our blood glucose.

You can find out the quantity of carbohydrate in foods pretty easily—it's usually on the packaging, or you can look in one of those little food counter books. Making a decision about carbohydrate quality, however, can be guesswork. The old complex-versus-simple-carbohydrate approach doesn't tell the true story.

What will tell you something about carbohydrate 'quality' is a food's GI. We discuss the GI in more detail later in this chapter, for now all you need to know is that the GI is just a number (actually it is a ranking) that reflects the glycaemic potential of carbohydrates: their ability to raise your blood glucose levels. Depending on the source of the carbohydrates (i.e. the actual food as prepared and eaten), they can raise blood glucose levels quite a lot, or just a little.

Healthy low GI foods are the key to unlocking the benefits of *The New Glucose Revolution* and achieving weight loss, blood glucose control and lifelong health. If you make the change and base your diet around eating balanced low GI meals, you will achieve lower insulin levels, making it easier for your body to burn fat and less likely that fat will be stored in all those places you don't want it.

Unlike a low carbohydrate diet, eating the low GI way is healthy, balanced and safe for children and adults alike. Not only that, it helps you expand your healthy eating choices, lose weight, feel fuller and manage many of your PCOS symptoms all at the same time.

The GI—and its newer companion value, the glycaemic load (GL)—are relevant *not just to you* but also your family. People with a family history of obesity, diabetes and heart disease gain the most from putting the GI into practice. It's ideal for those who want to do the best they can to prevent these problems in the first place.

In this chapter we cover the scientific rationale of healthy low GI eating. We also look at metabolism and the fuel hierarchy; why we need carbohydrates; how much you need; and how understanding the GI can help you choose the right amount of carbohydrates and the right type for managing PCOS.

GI low **GI medium** **or** **GI high**	Watch out for GI symbols on foods. In the UK, products are starting to be labelled—a number of major supermarket chains are in the process of testing and labelling their foods. A GI symbol or label is your guarantee that the GI value on the label is correct (it's been tested properly by an accredited laboratory). Visit the website for more details: www.glycemicindex.com

Healthy low GI eating is for everybody,
every day, every meal.

PCOS and the insulin connection

If you have PCOS, your body has a hard time bringing blood glucose levels down after you've eaten. PCOS means the body is insensitive, or you could say partially deaf, to insulin. The organs and tissues that ought to respond to even a small rise in insulin remain unresponsive. So, the body tries harder, by secreting even more insulin, to achieve the same effect, pretty much the way we all tend to raise our voice for someone who is hard of hearing. Thus high insulin levels are part and parcel of insulin resistance.

We now know that any means of improving insulin sensitivity, including drugs and weight loss, will improve symptoms of PCOS. Many doctors have found that low GI diets are particularly useful for women with PCOS. In addition, research is showing that low GI diets improve weight loss and appetite control.

Low GI diets have been proven to reduce blood glucose levels in people with diabetes. Just like women with PCOS, most people with diabetes are severely insulin resistant. If glucose levels come down in diabetes, then it's likely a low GI diet will bring down both glucose and insulin levels in anyone with insulin resistance.

Low GI diets are consistent with all the other dietary changes needed for preventing diabetes, heart disease and cancer, so you have nothing to lose and much to gain by following a safe, balanced and healthy low GI eating plan.

What you need to know about your metabolism and the fuel hierarchy

Our bodies run on fuel, just like a car runs on petrol. The fuels our bodies burn are derived from a mixture of the protein, fat, carbohydrate and alcohol that we consume. Every day we need to fill our fuel tanks with the right amount and the right kind of fuel for health, energy and to feel our best. The actual proportions in our fuel mix will vary from hour to hour and are determined to a large extent by the last meal we ate.

There's also a fuel 'hierarchy': an order of priority that our bodies follow for burning the fuels in food. Alcohol is at the top of the list because our bodies have no place to store unused alcohol (which is why it is a good idea to cut right back on alcohol if you need to lose weight). Protein comes second, followed by carbohydrate, while fat comes off last. In practice, the fuel mix is largely a combination of carbohydrate and fat in varying proportions. After meals the mix is predominantly carbohydrate and between meals it is mainly fat.

First of all let's focus on fat. The body's ability to burn all the fat we eat is one of the keys to weight control. If fat burning is inhibited, fat stores gradually accumulate. This is why the relative proportions of fat to carbohydrate in our fuel mix are critical. The proportions can vary throughout the day and are dictated by the level of insulin in the blood. For example, if our insulin levels are low, as they are when we first wake up in the morning, then the fuel mix is mainly fat. But, if our insulin levels are high, as they are after we have eaten a high carbohydrate meal then the fuel mix we burn is mainly carbohydrate.

However, if insulin is always high, as it is if you have PCOS, then your body is constantly forced to burn carbohydrate and has trouble burning the fat that is eaten and using it as a source of fuel. When this happens, fat stores mount up. Scientists now believe that subtle abnormalities in the ability to burn fat are behind most states of being overweight or obese.

Carbohydrate is nature's primary fuel

Did you know that carbohydrate is the most widely consumed substance in the world after water? In fact, carbohydrates hold a very special place in human nutrition.

THE PANCREAS PRODUCES INSULIN

The pancreas is a vital organ near the stomach. Its job is to produce the hormone insulin. Carbohydrate stimulates the secretion of insulin more than any other component of food including protein and fat. The slow absorption of the carbohydrate in low GI foods means that the pancreas doesn't have to work so hard and produces less insulin. If the pancreas is overstimulated over a long period of time, it may become 'exhausted', resulting in gestational diabetes and/or type 2 diabetes—both are common in women with a history of PCOS. Even without diabetes, high insulin levels are undesirable because they increase the risk of weight gain and heart disease.

Glucose, the simplest carbohydrate, is the *essential* fuel for the human brain, red blood cells and a growing foetus, and the main source of energy for our muscles during strenuous exercise. So it makes no sense to leave it out altogether. Low carb diets are unnecessarily restrictive and likely to reduce your short-term mental and physical performance. They may also cause heart disease and cancer long term.

Top 20 sources of carbohydrate

While sources of carbohydrate differ from country to country, most women in developed nations get their carbs from the same types of foods. A study in the United States in 2002 (the Harvard Nurses' Health Study) that looked at the diet of more than 120 000 nurses found that the top 20 sources of carbohydrate in their diet were:

1. Potato
2. White bread
3. Breakfast cereal
4. Dark bread (wholegrain or rye)
5. Orange juice
6. Banana
7. White rice
8. Pizza
9. Pasta
10. Muffin/cake
11. Fruit drink
12. Soft drink
13. Apple
14. Skimmed milk
15. Pancake
16. Table sugar
17. Jam
18. Fruit juice
19. French fries
20. Candy/confectionery

What is carbohydrate?

Carbohydrate is simply a part of food. It is the starchy part of foods like rice, bread, potatoes and pasta. It is also the ingredient that makes foods taste sweet: the sugars in fruit and honey are carbohydrates, as are the refined sugars in soft drinks and sweets.

Carbohydrate comes mainly from plant foods, such as cereal grains, fruits, vegetables and legumes (peas and beans). Milk products contain carbohydrate in the form of milk sugar or lactose. Lactose is the first carbohydrate we encounter as infants, and our human milk contains more lactose than any other mammal milk. It accounts for almost half the energy available to the infant.

Some foods contain a large amount of carbohydrate (cereals, potatoes, legumes and corn are good examples), while other foods, such as string beans, broccoli and salad greens, have very small amounts of carbohydrate. You can eat the latter freely, but they can't provide anywhere near enough carbohydrate for a moderate carbohydrate diet. And as nutritious as they can be, plain green salads aren't meals by themselves and should be complemented by a carbohydrate-dense food such as bread or legumes.

The following foods are high in carbohydrate and provide very little fat. Include them regularly in your eating plan, but spare the butter, margarine and oil when you prepare them.

Cereal grains

These include rice, wheat, oats, barley, rye and anything made from them (bread, pasta, breakfast cereal and flour). Low GI, wholegrain types are the best choices.

Fruits

A few tasty examples are apples, oranges, bananas, grapes and peaches.

Starchy vegetables

Foods such as corn, taro and sweet potato help to create filling, satisfying, low GI meals.

Legumes

Baked beans, lentils, kidney beans and chickpeas are excellent low GI choices.

Milk

Not only is milk a source of carbohydrate, recent studies suggest that the calcium in dairy foods helps weight control as well as insulin resistance. Reduced fat milks are the best choice.

As we explained, carbohydrate is a part of food. The following list will give you an idea how much carbohydrate there is in some popular foods.

Percentage of carbohydrate (grams per 100 grams of food) in food as eaten

apple 12%	orange 8%
baked beans 11%	pasta 70%
banana 21%	peas 8%
barley 61%	pear 12%
bread 47%	plum 6%
carrot 6%	potato 15%
cornflakes 85%	raisins 75%
cucumber 2%	rice 79%
flour 73%	split peas 45%
grapes 15%	sugar 100%
ice-cream 22%	sweet potato 17%
milk 5%	sweetcorn 16%
onion 5%	water cracker 71%
oats 61%	wheat biscuit 62%

Carbohydrate is brain food

Unlike our muscle cells, which can burn either fat or carbohydrate, our brain does not have the 'metabolic machinery' to burn fat. Unless we are literally starving (and we aren't just talking about skipping a meal or feeling very hungry here), carbohydrate is the only source of fuel that our brains can use. The brain is our most energy-demanding organ—responsible for over half our energy requirements in the resting state.

If you fast for 24 hours or decide not to eat carbohydrate at all, your brain will rely initially on small stores of carbohydrate in your liver. But within a few hours these will be depleted and your liver will begin synthesising glucose from non-carbohydrate sources (including your muscle tissue). It has only a limited ability to do this, however, and any shortfall in glucose availability will have consequences for your brain function and intellectual performance.

We know from some new studies that people perform demanding mental tasks better after eating a glucose load or carbohydrate-rich food. The mental tasks in the studies included various standard measures of 'intelligence' including word recall, maze learning, arithmetic, short-term memory, rapid information processing and reasoning. The young people, university students, people with diabetes, healthy elderly people and people with Alzheimer's disease who took part in the studies all showed improved mental ability following a carbohydrate meal.

At all times our bodies need to maintain a minimum threshold level of glucose in the blood to serve the brain and central nervous system. If for some reason glucose levels fall below this threshold (a state called 'hypoglycemia'), the consequences are severe, including trembling; dizziness; nausea; incoherent rambling speech; and lack of coordination. If not rectified, continuing hypoglycemia can lead to coma and even death. While such serious symptoms won't affect the average person, they are an ever present risk for people taking insulin or drugs to control high blood glucose levels.

What's wrong with a low carbohydrate diet?

Low carbohydrate diets are getting lots of attention these days. Finally, we are seeing scientific studies to determine whether they work or not and what effects they may have on your long-term health. Two recent ones showed that overweight people lost weight two to three times faster on a low carbohydrate diet than on a high carbohydrate one. Furthermore, there were no obvious adverse effects over a

When I passed a really important exam at my ballet school, my family and I decided we'd all go out to a club in town to celebrate. I hadn't eaten much that day as I had been really busy, just a slice of toast with peanut butter at lunchtime. My sister and I sneaked a small drink before we left and then at the club I probably overdid it— I had six gin cocktails over two hours. I don't remember snacking while I was drinking. The next thing I do remember is waking up in the emergency department of the local hospital, with an intravenous line delivering 5 per cent glucose. I had passed out in the club and was 'unresponsive'. The ambulance crew found my blood glucose drawn from a finger prick was really low (less than 2 mmol /L). The next day I was discharged apparently no worse for wear and told to go and see my local doctor who referred me to an endocrinologist because of the low blood glucose. The doctor asked me lots of questions and I recalled feeling a bit light-headed and sweaty on a few occasions in recent months. All the tests, however, showed nothing unusual at all. That's when the endocrinologist suggested to Mum and I that as a long shot he would check me out for PCOS (which I had never heard of) as a possible underlying cause of insulin resistance. This time the tests came up trumps. It was such a relief to find out what the matter was. I was prescribed metformin and put on a diet plan of healthy low GI eating including lots of vegetables, pasta, wholegrain bread and legumes. And, of course, was advised not to drink too much alcohol and, if I am out having a drink with friends, to make sure I have something to eat. I have to say I have become a real enthusiast for my new diet and I haven't missed a single dose of metformin. After two and a half years, despite a very active social life, I haven't experienced another episode of symptomatic low blood glucose which apparently is as rare as hen's teeth.

Melissa, 18

six-month period. However, people found it hard to stick to such restrictive diets and they eventually regained the weight they lost. So all that effort was wasted.

There's a lesson here too—high carbohydrate diets may not be the optimal way to lose weight. If they raise people's blood glucose and insulin levels, then it's no surprise that burning body fat will be twice as hard. Low carbohydrate diets may be effective in the short term because they lower glucose and insulin levels.

There are real concerns with low carbohydrate diets. They may help lower insulin levels temporarily, but their high saturated fat content may be causing lots of ill effects in the longer term. Indeed, high levels of saturated fats are un-equivocally associated with heart disease and heart attack.

For the first half of the last century, people with diabetes were told to follow low carbohydrate diets (to keep their blood glucose levels down) and to get their calories from high protein fatty foods. Trouble was, they were dying early of heart attack, rather than diabetes.

When cautious studies were carried out with high carbohydrate diets, doctors were stunned to find that blood glucose control improved and blood fats came down. Nowadays, after much research, people with diabetes are advised to follow a moderately high carbohydrate diet.

Most people also find low carbohydrate diets are hard to live with because they cut out so many of the foods that we love: bread, fruit, potatoes, pasta, to name just a few. It's not so surprising that people lose weight on such a limited diet. And it's even less surprising that they find it hard to stick to. Women with PCOS need to take a long-term view of their health—it's not just a few weeks of weight loss but a whole new way of eating to reduce your chances of developing diabetes or heart disease.

For weight control—not just in the short term but

keeping it off for good—you need to follow an eating plan that you love.

The bottom line is that the *type* of carbohydrate and the type of fat are more critical than the precise *amount*. Choosing low GI carbs will not only promote weight control, it will reduce blood glucose and insulin levels throughout the day, increase your sense of feeling full and satisfied, and provide bulk and a rich supply of micro-nutrients including zinc, calcium and magnesium. All these factors work together to increase insulin sensitivity and improve the signs and symptoms of PCOS.

> **Unlike low carbohydrate diets, low GI diets are safe, balanced and provide all the micronutrients for optimum health.**

How much carbohydrate do we need?

As we have shown, there are good reasons to avoid a low carbohydrate diet (less than 30 per cent of energy as carbs), but what then is the optimal level of carbohydrate in the diet? Should it be as high as 65 per cent of total daily calories, as some nutritionists and doctors recommend, or a more moderate 45 per cent of energy?

The American Institute of Medicine published new nutritional guidelines recently. Their recommendations indicate that both moderate and high levels (45–65 per cent of energy) or anything in between can work to meet the body's daily energy and nutritional needs while minimising the risk for chronic disease. In the UK, our dietary guidelines are being reviewed with a view to adopting the same flexible recommendations. And if we look carefully at diets around the world, it's clear that both high and moderate intakes of carbohydrate are commensurate with good health. The only group of people who naturally follow a low carbohydrate diet are traditional living Eskimos (Inuits), who eat large amounts of protein and unsaturated fat from seafood.

Our approach in *The Low GI Guide to Managing PCOS* and other titles in *The New Glucose Revolution* series is that your carbohydrate intake can be either high or moderate, as long as you give due consideration to the type of foods you eat. It may be helpful to discuss your own particular needs and food preferences with an accredited practising (a registered) dietitian (RD).

Is a high carbohydrate diet for you?

Most of the world's population currently eats a high carbo-hydrate diet based on staples such as rice, corn, millet and wheat-based foods like bread or noodles. In some African, Middle Eastern and Asian countries, for example, carbohy-drate may form as much as 70–80 per cent of a person's energy intake—but this is probably too high for optimum health. In contrast, people in industrialised nations such as the UK, United States, Australia and New Zealand eat less than half of their kilojoules (calories) as carbohydrates; typi-cally only 40–45 per cent carbohydrate. A high carbohydrate diet has more than 50 per cent of energy as carbohydrate.

Is consuming at least half of your total daily calories as carbohydrate realistic for you? That depends. If you have always been health conscious and avoided high fat foods, or if you enjoy an Asian-style diet most of the time, then chances are you're already eating a high carbohydrate diet.

Of course, the number of calories, and hence the amount of carbohydrate, varies with your weight and activity levels. If you are an active person with average energy require-ments who is not trying to lose weight (i.e. with an average intake of 2000 calories or 8400 kJ per day), you will eat

275 grams of carbohydrate. If you are trying to lose weight and are consuming a low kilojoule diet (i.e. a small eater on 1200 calories or 5000 kJ per day), it means eating about 165 grams of carbohydrate a day.

Is a moderate carbohydrate diet for you?

A Mediterranean-style diet that includes olive oil and nuts is higher in fat and provides only about 45 per cent of energy as carbohydrate. In the past, dietitians and nutritionists in countries like the UK, Australia, New Zealand and the US would have frowned upon this, but that's no longer the case. We now know that as long as you carefully consider the types of fats and the types of carbohydrate, then this amount of carbohydrate is perfectly compatible with good health. At this level, you need to consume at least 125 grams of carbohydrate a day if you are a small eater and 225 grams if you are an average eater.

> Today's health recommendations are as much about the type of fat and the nature of the carbohydrate as about the total amounts of each.

In the end, the choice of how much carbohydrate you eat—moderate or high—is yours. Our approach has built-in flexibility when it comes to the amount of carbohydrate you need to eat. It's not rocket science to suggest that the way of eating that you'll enjoy and tend to follow over the long term is the one that is closest to your usual diet and to your cultural and ethnic origins. What we emphasise is that the *type* or *source* of the carbohydrate and fat are just as important as the amount. We believe that, unlike baseball caps, one size does not fit all.

The GI: the real deal on carbohydrate

It's time to look at the type or nature of the carbohydrate in your diet. The most important thing to keep in mind is that all carbohydrates were not created equal—you must choose the right kind of carbohydrate for your lifestyle.

Traditionally, the nature of carbohydrates was described by their chemical structure: simple or complex. Sugars were simple and starches were complex, simply because sugars were small molecules and starches were big. By virtue of their large size, it was automatically assumed that complex carbohydrates, such as starches, would be slowly digested and absorbed by our bodies and would cause only a small and gradual rise in blood glucose levels. Simple sugars, on the other hand, were assumed to be the villains of the piece, being digested and absorbed quickly, producing a rapid rise in blood glucose.

HOW TO FIND A DIETITIAN

For specific information about your own kilojoule and exact carbohydrate needs, you should consult a registered dietitian (RD). For a list of registered dietitians, visit the website www.bda.uk.com. Alternatively, send a self-addressed envelope to the British Dietetic Association (BDA), in order to receive a list of registered dietitians. The list will have the RD names, locations and telephone numbers. The address of the BDA is: 5th Floor Charles House, 148/9 Great Charles Street, Queens Way, Birmingham, B3 3HT.

In addition, the following website provides specific information about dietitians specialising in the GI: www.diagnosemefirst.com.

Make sure that the person you choose has the letters RD after his or her name.

A few very elementary experiments long ago on raw starches and pure sugars seemed to support these assumptions, and for 50 years they were taught to every medical and biochemistry student as 'fact'.

We now know that the whole chemical concept of 'simple' versus 'complex' carbohydrate does not tell us anything about how the carbohydrates in our food change blood glucose levels in our bodies. Twenty years of scientific research with real people and real food have shown that those assumptions about the speed of digestion were all wrong.

The rise in blood glucose after meals could not be predicted simply on the basis of a simple versus complex chemical structure. Another system of describing the nature of carbohydrates and classifying them according to their effects on blood glucose was needed: the glycaemic index or GI as it is now widely known, served that purpose.

It may seem surprising today, but scientists did not study the actual blood glucose responses to common foods in real people until the early 1980s. Since 1981, hundreds of different foods have been tested as single foods and in mixed meals with both healthy people and people with diabetes. Professors David Jenkins and Tom Wolever at the University of Toronto were the first to introduce the term 'glycaemic index' to compare the ability of different carbohydrates to raise blood glucose levels.

The glycaemic index or GI is simply a numerical way of describing how the carbohydrates in individual foods affect blood glucose levels. Foods with a high GI value contain carbohydrates that cause a dramatic rise in blood glucose levels, while foods with a low GI value contain carbohydrates with much less impact. This research has turned some widely held beliefs upside down.

The GI is a measure of how fast
carbohydrates hit the bloodstream.
It compares carbohydrates weight for
weight, gram for gram.

The first surprise was that the starch in foods like bread, potatoes and many types of rice is digested and absorbed very quickly, not slowly, as had always been assumed.

Second, scientists found that the sugar in foods (like fruit, confectionery and ice-cream) did not produce more rapid or prolonged rises in blood glucose, as had always been thought. The truth was that most of the sugars in foods, regardless of the source, actually produced quite moderate blood glucose responses, lower than most starches.

So we all need to forget the old distinctions that have been made between starchy foods and sugary foods, or simple versus complex carbohydrates. They have no useful application when it comes to blood glucose levels. Even an experienced scientist with a detailed knowledge of a food's chemical composition finds it difficult to predict a food's GI value.

Forget about the words simple and
complex carbohydrate.
Think in terms of low and high GI values.

The key to understanding the GI is the rate of digestion

Foods containing carbohydrates that break down quickly during digestion have the highest GI values. The blood glucose response is fast and high. In other words, the glucose (or sugar) in the bloodstream increases rapidly. Conversely, foods that contain carbohydrates that break down slowly, releasing glucose gradually into the bloodstream, have a low GI value.

An analogy we like to use is the popular fable of the tortoise and the hare. The hare, just like high GI foods, speeds away but loses the race to the tortoise with his slow and steady pace. Similarly, slow and steady low GI foods produce a smooth blood glucose curve without wild fluctuations. The graph below shows the different effects of slow and fast carbohydrates on our blood glucose levels.

For most people, foods with low GI values have advantages over those with high GI values; however, in elite sport, there are times when a high GI food will be the best choice.

The substance that produces one of the greatest effects

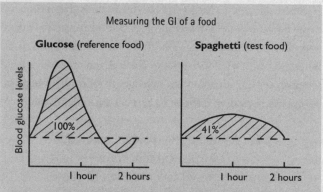

Measuring the GI of a food

Glucose (reference food)   **Spaghetti** (test food)

The test food and the reference food must contain the same amount of carbohydrate. The usual dose is 50 grams but sometimes 25 grams is used when the portion size would be otherwise too large. Even smaller doses such as 15 grams have been used. The GI result is much the same whatever the dose because the GI is simply a relative measure of carbohydrate quality.

on blood glucose levels is pure glucose itself. GI testing has shown that most foods have less effect on blood glucose levels than glucose (also called dextrose). The GI value of pure glucose is set at 100 and every other food is ranked on a scale from 0 to 100 according to the actual effect on blood glucose levels. (Note: There are a few foods that have GI values of more than 100, e.g. jasmine rice. While this seems extraordinary, there's a simple explanation. Glucose is a highly concentrated solution that tends to be held up briefly in the stomach. On the other hand, jasmine rice contains starch that leaves the stomach without delay and is then digested at lightning speed.)

> The glycaemic index is a clinically proven tool
> in its applications to diabetes and weight control.

What determines a food's GI?

Everyone wants to know what gives one food a high GI value and another one a low GI value. There is a wealth of information, which can easily confuse. We have summarised in simple terms the results of the most recent scientific research in the table on pages 55–56 which looks at the various factors that influence the GI value of a food.

The key message is that the physical state of the starch in a food is by far the most important factor influencing its GI value. That's why the advances in food processing over the past 200 years have had such a profound effect on the overall GI values of the carbohydrates we eat.

The GI was never meant to be used in isolation!

At first glance when you look at a list of foods with a low GI value it might appear that some high fat foods such as chocolate seem a good choice simply because they have a low GI value. This is absolutely not the case. A food's GI value was never meant to be the only criterion by which it

DIGESTING CARBOHYDRATES

To make use of the sugars and starches in foods, our bodies first have to break them down into a form that we can absorb and that our bodies can use. This is what we call digestion.

Digestion starts in the mouth where the starch-digesting enzyme in our saliva which is called amylase, is incorporated into our food as we chew. Amylase chops up long-chain starch molecules into short-chain molecules such as maltose and maltodextrins. Its activity is halted by the acids secreted into the stomach and most digestion continues only when the carbohydrate leaves the stomach and reaches the small intestine.

The rate at which food enters the small intestine from the stomach is called the rate of stomach (or gastric) emptying. Some food components—such as viscous or 'sticky' fibre, acidic compounds such as vinegar, and very concentrated solutions—help to slow down stomach emptying and therefore the overall speed of carbohydrate digestion.

In the small intestine, starch digestion continues. Huge amounts of amylase are secreted in pancreatic juice into the small intestine, so much so that the biochemists call it amylase 'overkill'. The speed of digestion now depends on the nature of the starch itself—how resistant it is in a physical and chemical sense to being attacked by enzymes. Many starches in food are rapidly digested, while others are more resistant and the process is slower.

Other food factors may influence the speed of digestion. If the mixture of food and enzymes is highly viscous or sticky, owing to the presence of viscous fibre, mixing slows down and the enzymes and starch take longer to make contact. The products of starch digestion will also take longer to move toward the wall of the intestine, where the last steps in digestion take place.

At the intestinal wall, the short-chain starch products, together with the sugars in foods, are broken down by specific enzymes. The monosaccharides that finally result from starch and sugar digestion include glucose, fructose and galactose. They are absorbed from the small intestine into the bloodstream, where they are available as a source of energy to the cells.

is judged. Large amounts of fat (and protein) in food tend to slow the rate of stomach emptying and therefore the rate at which foods are digested in the small intestine.

High fat foods will therefore tend to have lower GI values than their low fat equivalents. For example, potato chips have a lower GI value (54) than boiled, new (78). Many biscuits have a lower GI value (40-60) than some breads, for example white bread (70). In these instances, a lower GI value doesn't mean an automatically better choice from a nutritional standpoint. Saturated fat in these foods will have adverse effects on coronary health, far greater than the benefit of lower blood glucose levels. These foods should be treated as 'indulgences'.

This is not to say that all fats in foods should be avoided. One of the reasons why nuts have such a low GI value is their relatively high fat content compared to cereal grains. But just as there are differences in the nature of carbohydrates in foods, there are differences in the quality of fats. We need to be choosy about fats too. Healthy fats, such as the omega-3 polyunsaturated fats, are not only good for us, they help to lower the blood glucose response to meals.

The right kind of carbohydrate

Both high and moderate carbohydrate intake can be healthy—the choice is simply up to you. Both types of diets,

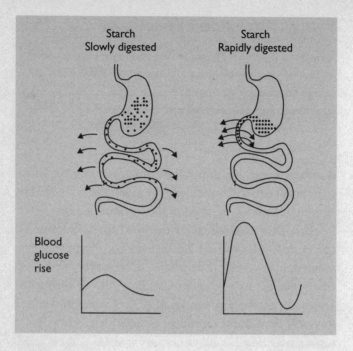

however, need to emphasise low GI carbohydrates and healthy fats.

To ensure that you are eating enough carbohydrate and the right kind, you should eat:

- fruits for snacks or dessert: aim for 4–5 pieces per day

- vegetables with lunch and dinner and even as snacks: aim for at least five serves per day

- at least one low GI food at each meal: aim for four serves of wholegrain cereals per day

- lots of fibre (foods with low energy density or fewer calories per gram)

Factors that influence the GI value of a food

FACTOR	MECHANISM	EXAMPLES OF FOOD WHERE THE EFFECT IS SEEN
Starch gelatinisation	The less gelatinised (swollen) the starch, the slower the rate of digestion.	Al dente spaghetti, oatmeal and biscuits have less gelatinised starch.
Physical entrapment	The fibrous coat around beans and seeds and plant cell walls acts as a physical barrier, slowing down access of enzymes to the starch inside.	Pumpernickel and grainy bread, legumes and barley.
High amylose to amylopectin ratio*	The more amylose a food contains, the less water the starch will absorb and the slower its rate of digestion.	Basmati rice and legumes contain more amylose than other cereals.
Particle size	The smaller the particle size, the easier it is for water and enzymes to penetrate.	Finely milled flours have high GI values. Stone ground flours have larger particles and lower GIs.
Viscosity of fibre	Viscous, soluble fibres increase the viscosity of the intestinal contents and this slows down the interaction between the starch and the enzymes.	Finely milled wholemeal and rye flours have fast rates of digestion and absorption because the fibre is not fibrous. Rolled oats, beans, lentils and apples.
Sugar	The digestion of sugar produces only half as many glucose molecules as the same amount of starch (the other half is fructose). The presence of sugar also restricts gelatinisation of the starch by binding water and reducing the amount of 'available' water.	Morning Coffee™ biscuits, oatmeal biscuits and some breakfast cereals (Kellogg's® Frosties®) that are high in sugar have relatively low GI values.

Factors that influence the GI value of a food (*cont.*)

FACTOR	MECHANISM	EXAMPLES OF FOOD WHERE THE EFFECT IS SEEN
Acidity	Acids in food slow down stomach emptying, thereby slowing the rate at which starch can be digested.	Vinegar, lemon juice, lime juice, some salad dressings, pickled vegetables, and sourdough bread.
Fat	Fat slows down the rate of stomach emptying, thereby slowing the digestion of the starch.	Potato chips have a lower GI value than boiled white potatoes.

* Amylose and amylopectin are two different types of starch. Both are found in foods, but the ratio varies.

THE EFFECT OF STARCH GELATINISATION ON THE GLYCAEMIC INDEX

The starch in raw food is stored in hard, compact granules that make it difficult to digest. Most starchy foods need to be cooked for this reason. During cooking, water and heat expand the starch granules to different degrees; some granules actually burst and the individual starch molecules release. This process is called gelatinisation.

The swollen granules and free starch molecules are very easy to digest. The quick action of the enzymes results in a rapid, high blood glucose rise after consumption. A food containing starch that is fully gelatinised will therefore have a very high GI value.

GLYCAEMIC LOAD

Glycaemic load provides a measure of the degree of glycemia and insulin demand produced by a normal serving of the food.

Glycaemic load is calculated simply by multiplying the GI of a food by the amount of carbohydrate per serving and dividing by 100.

Glycaemic load = (GI × carbohydrate per serving) ÷ 100.

The glycaemic load is greatest for those foods which provide the most carbohydrate, particularly those we tend to eat in large quantities. Some nutritionists have argued that the glycaemic load is an improvement on the GI because it provides an estimate of both quantity and quality of carbohydrate (the GI gives us just quality). In large scale studies however, the risk of disease is often linked to the GI but not to the glycaemic load. It appears that more carbohydrate is better than less, especially from low GI food sources.

Don't make the mistake of using GL alone. If you do, you might find yourself eating a diet with very little carbohydrate but a lot of fat, especially saturated fat, and excessive amounts of protein. Use the glycaemic index to compare foods of similar nature (e.g. bread with bread) and use the glycaemic load with caution.

You'll find both the GI and GL of many foods in the tables on pages 189–203. For more comprehensive tables please refer to *The Low GI Shopper's Guide to GI values*.

You will find that when you are choosy about your carbohydrate, your insulin levels will be lower and you will automatically burn more fat. You may not feel this change as it is happening, but you will see the results over time (you'll lose weight!) Eating high fibre foods will also help fill you up and prevent you overeating.

The right kind of fat

For most people, 'low fat' is still synonymous with 'healthy' and 'weight loss'. Forget it! Once upon a time, when fruits, vegetables and wholegrains were the staples of a low fat diet, it might have been true. But it is no longer so—indeed, the typical low fat diet may be distinctly unhealthy and one of the reasons behind our expanding waistlines. In the 1990s, the experts told us to eat low fat diets because they were concerned about two things. First, saturated fat increases the risk of heart disease; second, fatty foods are too easily over-eaten because they are energy-dense. Those concerns are still valid today. But the solution to the problem—recommending a low fat diet—has not been a successful strategy. While we've cut down on total fat, we haven't cut down on saturated fat, and the food industry (with the best intentions) gave us a myriad low fat foods that were just as energy-dense as their full fat counterparts. So during the 1990s, the era of '99% fat free', the prevalence of obesity soared, and with it heart disease and diabetes.

As a result of these unexpected events, the British Heart Foundation went back to the drawing board and remodelled their dietary advice. Now the message is: first, the type of fat is more important for health than the total amount, and second, the energy density of a food (calories or kilojoules per serve) is more important to weight control than the fat content.

Furthermore, most of us need to eat *more* of certain kinds of fat for optimal health (yes, you read it right). These include the omega-3 fats found in fish, canola-based products and omega-3 enriched eggs. Eating these and more monounsaturated fats like those in olive oil and canola oil has been shown to significantly reduce the risk of a heart attack. Indeed, one of the most important diet studies ever carried out, the Lyon Heart study, showed that this type of diet (with more fish, fruit, vegies and good fats) was twice as effective in reducing the risk of another heart attack as the standard low fat diet recommended by the American Heart Association.

There's another excellent reason why you should aim to increase these fats at the expense of the saturated ones. While all fats have the same number of calories or kilojoules per gram, they may not all have the same effect on your weight. For reasons that are not yet clear, a weight loss diet which emphasises fish or monounsaturated fats like olive oil is much more likely to reduce abdominal body fat. This is a critical point for women with PCOS whose excess fat around the waist is directly linked to their insulin resistance. If they can reduce that stubborn fat, insulin levels will come down and hence reduce signs and symptoms of PCOS.

Where do you find the good fats?

- fish such as salmon, tuna, herrings, sardines—canned or fresh—but any fish is better than none at all

- shellfish, prawns, scallops

- walnuts, almonds, cashews—best unsalted, forget the chips and salty snacks

- avocado—spread it on bread as an alternative to margarine or butter

- olives—spread as a tapenade or add whole to almost anything—pasta sauces or salads

- muesli—mix sunflower seeds, pumpkin seeds, ground almond or hazelnuts

- linseed is a great source of omega-3 fats: try soya and linseed bread

There are two important things to remember in improving your diet:

1. Identify the sources of carbohydrate in your diet and reduce high GI foods. Don't go to extremes; there is room for your favourite high GI foods.

2. Identify the sources of fat and look at ways you can reduce saturated fat. Choose monounsaturated and polyunsaturated fats, such as olive oil and sunflower oil, instead of saturated fats like butter and shortening. Again, don't go overboard—the body needs some fat, and there's room for your favourite fatty foods on occasion.

What about protein?

Incorporating more protein in our diet makes good sense for weight control. Protein is tops in terms of satiety—that pleasant feeling of fullness after eating. In comparison with carbohydrate and fat, protein makes us feel more satisfied immediately after eating and reduces hunger between meals. That's critically important because hunger makes or breaks a diet and compromises long-term weight control. Protein also increases our metabolic rate during the hour or two after eating. We burn more energy by the minute compared with the increase that occurs after eating carbs or fats. Even though this is a relatively small difference it may be important in long-term weight control. Lastly, protein foods are excellent sources of micronutrients, such as iron, zinc, vitamin B12 and omega-3 fats. So, even though you're cutting energy intake, you're not cutting good nutrition.

Most of us obtain about 15 per cent of the energy in our diet from protein. If you wish (it's up to you) you can increase this to as much as 30 per cent without cause for concern. Recent studies show that this higher level increases the rate of weight and body fat loss, at least in the short term. In a similar way to carbohydrate and fat, the *source* of extra protein is critical. Lean meats (beef, pork, lamb), chicken, fish and shellfish are ideal. Go for the leanest cuts in the supermarket—grill, stir-fry or barbecue, and cut off all the visible fat.

Dairy products are more than good sources of protein—the combination of protein and calcium that's unique to dairy appears to aid weight control. Studies have shown that the more calcium or dairy (it's hard to separate the two) people eat, the lower their weight and fat mass. Calcium is known to be intimately involved in the burning of fat—and that's something we want to encourage! However, we have to be a little selective about which dairy foods we eat. Choose low fat dairy products including milk, yoghurt and cheese.

Nuts are also excellent sources of protein and micro-nutrients too but we have to be careful not to overdo them—they are very energy-dense and pack a lot of kilojoules into a small weight.

Finally, eggs are great sources of protein and essential vitamins and minerals. If you select the 'omega-3' eggs on the market, you will also boost the good fats in your diet.

Not all carbohydrates were created equal—
you must choose the right kind of carbohydrate
for your lifestyle.

Summing up

Let's sum up the main points we've covered in this chapter.

- There are sound reasons to eat a moderately high carbohydrate diet if you have PCOS.

- Low carb diets are unnecessarily restrictive and may be harmful in the long term.

- The nature of the carbohydrate is more important than the absolute amount.

- Low GI carbs lower insulin levels and improve insulin sensitivity, the key to beating PCOS.

- Low GI carbs are more satiating and help reduce hunger between meals, the key to long-term weight control.

- The kind of fat is more important than the amount: reduce saturated fat, increase the good fats.

- Higher protein intake may be helpful to weight control.

In the next chapter, we show you exactly what you need to do and eat to put it all into practice.

IS IT LOW, MEDIUM, OR HIGH? THE GI OF SOME POPULAR CARB FOODS AT A GLANCE

A **low** GI value is 55 or less.

A **moderate/medium** GI value is 56 to 69 inclusive.

A **high** GI value is 70 or more.

The GI ratings in this table are based on the average of tested foods. See the GI values tables on page 189 for more details. Foods high in saturated fat are indicated ■.

FRUIT AND VEGETABLES

Fruit: All fruits contain carbohydrate from their natural sugar content and most have a low or medium GI. Temperate climate fruits—apples, pears, citrus and stone fruits all have low GI values. Tropical fruits— cantaloupe, pineapple, paw paw, papaya and watermelon—tend to have higher GI values, but their glycaemic load (GL) is low because they are low in carbohydrate.

	GI
Apples	low
Bananas	low
Berries (all)	low
Grapefruit	low
Grapes	low
Mangoes	low
Oranges	low
Peaches	low
Pears	low
Plums	low
Cantaloupe	medium
Cherries	medium
Kiwi fruit	medium
Paw Paw	medium
Pineapple	medium
Watermelon	high

Vegetables: Apart from starchy vegetables, most vegetables have very little carbohydrate so do not have a GI value. Think of green vegetables from asparagus and broccoli to spinach and courgette and all salad vegetables as 'free' foods that are full of fibre, essential nutrients and protective anti-oxidants that will fill you up without adding extra kilojoules. Some vegetables like carrots, peas, parsnip and pumpkin have very little carb in the amounts normally eaten so eat and enjoy.

	GI
Carrots	low
Green peas	low
Sweetcorn	low
Sweet potato	low
Taro	low
Yam	low
Beetroot, canned	medium
*Potato, baby new canned	medium
Broad beans	high
Parsnip	high
*Potato	high
Pumpkin	high
Swede	high

* What about potatoes? Potatoes generally have a high GI. If you love them, try and replace some potato with low GI starchy vegetables. And when you do choose potato, look for varieties such as baby new potatoes, which have a lower GI.

BREADS AND CEREALS

Cereal grains (rice, wheat, oats, barley and rye) and products made from them (bread, breakfast cereals, flour, pasta and noodles, biscuits and cakes etc) are the most concentrated sources of carbohydrate in our diet so have a major impact on the overall GI of our diet. Wholegrain breads and cereals have many health benefits and most have a lower GI than refined cereal grains. Look for the low GI label on commercial breads and breakfast cereals.

THE LOW GI GUIDE TO MANAGING PCOS

Bread	GI
Chapati (with besan or barley flour)	low
Fruit loaf	low
Grainy and granary breads	low
Sourdough bread	low
Soya and linseed bread	low
Wholegrain bread	low
Croissant	medium
Crumpet	medium
Pita bread	medium
Pumpernickel	medium
Rye bread	medium
Bagel	high
White bread	high
Wholemeal bread	high

Breakfast cereals	
All-Bran®	low
Muesli	low
Porridge oats (not instant)	low
Toasted muesli ■	low
Corn flakes	high
Porridge (instant)	high

Cereal grains, pasta, rice and noodles	
Barley	low
Buckwheat	low
Bulgur (burghul)	low
Buckwheat	low
Noodles – cellophane	low
– instant	low
– rice	low
– soba	low
Pasta, dried and fresh	low
Quinoa	low
Arborio rice	medium
Basmati rice	medium
Wild rice	medium
Udon noodles	medium
Instant rice	high
Jasmine rice	high
Spaghetti, canned in tomato sauce	high

LEGUMES INCLUDING BEANS, PEAS AND LENTILS

Whether you buy dried legumes and cook them yourself or convenient canned products including salad bean or pulse mixes you are choosing one of nature's lowest GI foods.

	GI		GI
Baked beans	low	Lentils – green	low
Black beans	low	– red	low
Black-eyed beans	low	Lima beans	low
Borlotti beans	low	Mung beans	low
Butter beans	low	Pinto beans	low
Cannellini beans	low	Romano beans	low
Chick peas (garbanzo beans)	low	Soya beans	low
Haricot/Navy beans	low	Split peas	low
Kidney beans	low		

DAIRY PRODUCTS AND ALTERNATIVES

Virtually all dairy foods have a low GI thanks to lactose, the sugar found naturally in milk, which has a GI of 46. Dairy foods are among the richest sources of calcium in our diet. Choose low fat dairy foods to reduce your saturated fat intake.

	GI		GI
Milk – Full fat ■	low	Yoghurt, low fat	low
– Skimmed	low	Ice-cream – Regular ■	low
Soya milk, calcium enriched, low fat	low	– Low fat	low
		Milk, condensed, sweetened ■	medium

Look for the GI label on the foods you buy

A number of major food companies and supermarket chains are progressively testing and labelling their foods. A GI symbol or label on the packet tells you that a food has been glycaemic index tested.

CHAPTER 3

TAKING CHARGE

Four steps to taking charge
Managing your weight
Avoiding the dreaded yoyo dieting cycle
So, what's the healthy way to lose weight?
Eating well
How do I change my diet?
Moving more with PCOS
What type of exercise and how much?
Our top ten ways to get moving
Building more activity into your day
How to stay motivated? That's not just *your* problem
Take care of yourself

When we talk to women with PCOS the one thing they tell us time and again is that they feel 'out of control'—gaining weight, being unable to fall pregnant, and growing an excessive amount of body hair in areas where it just shouldn't be. We have found that by showing these women how to make some basic lifestyle changes, such as eating the right kinds of food and exercising more, they can start to feel in control of their lives again. In fact, by following our diet and exercise suggestions many women have found that they can take charge of their health in a way they never have before, and can effectively manage their PCOS symptoms.

We started this book by describing, as simply as we could, what PCOS is, the insulin connection and why what you eat plays such an important part in helping you manage PCOS symptoms. It's time now to show you how you can make the change to low GI healthy eating and build more exercise into your life. This chapter is about the four steps to taking charge and is packed with plenty of practical ideas you can implement right now.

The real benefits we have seen with many women and girls who have adopted a healthy low GI way of eating and stepped up the exercise and activity schedule include:

- improving PCOS symptoms—regulating menstrual cycles, reducing acne and excess hair growth

- achieving and maintaining a healthy weight

- controlling blood glucose and insulin levels

- balancing hormone levels

- boosting fertility

- gaining control and quality of life

And, if pregnancy is one of your plans for the future, making these lifestyle changes can lead to dramatic improvements in ovulation, pregnancy rates and reducing the risk of miscarriage.

At the same time, you will also be going a long way towards reducing your risk of developing type 2 diabetes and heart disease.

By the way, when we use the word 'diet' we're talking about eating the healthy low GI way, not about those restrictive diets that we know don't work in the long term.

Four steps to taking charge

Be reassured, we aren't going to ask you to work out on a treadmill for hours on end, starve yourself, or try and remember long food lists of do's and don'ts. Quite the opposite. Our programme is based on little changes that you can easily incorporate into your life and that you will feel comfortable with. In addition, we can promise that you won't feel hungry and, if you stick to it, you'll have more energy. What's more, we don't expect you to do everything in one go. One step at a time is fine. The four basic steps to taking charge of your PCOS symptoms the healthy low GI way are:

- managing your weight

- eating the healthy low GI way

- moving more

- taking care of yourself

Managing your weight

Managing your weight is really important if you have PCOS. Being overweight increases insulin resistance, worsens the symptoms of PCOS and increases the risk of developing diabetes as you get older. The good news is that you don't need to lose a lot of weight (or body fat) to start improving your PCOS symptoms.

We now know from the women we have helped and from many scientific studies that losing as little as 5 per cent of body weight can help control blood glucose levels, improve menstrual function, reduce testosterone levels, improve an excess hair problem and help with acne. So how much weight does this actually mean? Well, if you are 100 kilograms (220 pounds) this means that losing around 5 kilograms (11 pounds) of body fat can make a difference, and if you are 70 kilograms (154 pounds) as little as 3.5 kilograms (8 pounds) can help you to start taking control. In the long term, you should aim to lose 10 per cent of your current body weight—this will go a long way towards reducing or even reversing your insulin resistance.

It makes sense that achieving and maintaining a healthy weight comes from balancing your energy intake from the food you eat with your energy output from whatever physical activity you do. So, when you take in more energy from food than you burn up, you tend to put on weight or, rather, store fat. To lose weight and shed that fat, you need to eat less or move more—and it's pretty obvious that the most effective way is to do a bit of both.

Here's the really important part: when we talk about eating less, we don't mean starving yourself and feeling hungry all the time. We mean choosing the right foods, the ones that the body burns rather than stores as fat and that satisfy the appetite for breakfast, lunch, dinner and snacks in between. So what are these seemingly miracle foods? Well, this is where the glycaemic index and eating the healthy low GI way comes in.

To whet your appetite, just imagine breakfasts such as barley porridge with dried fruit and yoghurt, wholemeal blueberry hotcakes, or sweetcorn, bacon and mushroom omelettes with wholegrain toast. Or main meals like pasta with roasted sweet potato and feta cheese, bean and corn burritos or lamb burgers. And for dessert there is cherry strudel, apple and rhubarb crumble with muesli and walnut topping or baked ricotta cheesecake? Hungry? You can enjoy all these foods and more when you take control and start managing your weight by eating well and moving more. In our experience, when women change to a healthy low GI diet they often comment on the fact that they are feeling fuller and are less tempted to snack on those 'not so healthy' energy-dense foods—a big help when you are trying to lose weight.

Avoiding the dreaded yoyo dieting cycle

If you want to lose body fat and keep it off, restrictive dieting isn't the answer. Calorie counting may help you lose 'weight' (on the scales), but doesn't necessarily help you lose body fat. And it's almost impossible for most people to stick to in the long term.

What happens when you go on a restrictive diet is that that you starve the body of carbohydrate, and use up the carbohydrate stores (glycogen) in the muscles. As every gram of glycogen is stored along with 3 grams of water, the initial fast drop in weight you see on the scales is mainly due to water loss. Once you have used up the glycogen stores in your muscles, the body breaks down some of its own muscle tissue to supply glucose to the brain. Lean muscle tissue, unlike fat, is active—it uses up energy even when you are at rest. Losing muscle tissue therefore slows down your metabolism, which means the body needs less energy to do the same work it used to. And this is how the dreaded yoyo dieting cycle begins.

EVER HEARD SOMEONE SAY 'I HAVE A SLOW METABOLISM', OR 'SHE'S LUCKY, SHE HAS A FAST METABOLISM'?

Here's what that really means. Your resting metabolic rate—the amount of energy you burn at rest—largely determines your ability to lose or gain weight. The lower your metabolic rate, the greater the tendency you have to gain weight. Your metabolic rate depends largely on the amount of muscle you have, so building muscle through exercise is an important part of weight control. Excessive dieting and overly restricting our food intake can reduce our metabolic rate. Eating the healthy low GI way and moving more help you to maintain a high metabolism. And that's important.

The human body is also extremely good at adapting to the amount of energy we give it and this is what happens when you starve your body with a restrictive diet. First your body tries to conserve energy, slowing down your metabolism. Then, as soon as you go off that restrictive diet (which, if you are like most people, is pretty inevitable), you will probably pile the weight you have just lost right back on, plus a bit extra because your body now needs less energy to survive than it used to. So, if you go on and off diets, your body ends up with less and less muscle and more and more fat, which is why restrictive dieting can make you fat.

In the end, most restrictive diets don't work because they are just too hard to stick to for any length of time. If you are hungry and tired all the time, or if what you have to eat on your restrictive diet doesn't fit in with your family and social life, you may see the weight drop off in the first few weeks, but you are unlikely to stick with the diet long term.

So, what's the healthy way to lose weight?

Here are some tips on the healthy way to help you lose weight and keep it off long term.

First of all, aim to lose body fat rather than weight. Put the scales away and get out the tape measure. It's more useful to go by how your clothes fit. If your body is fit and toned, who cares what it weighs?

Don't think about going on a restrictive diet. The only way to lose weight and body fat permanently is to change your eating habits and include regular physical activity in your day. This can mean changing the habits of a lifetime, so don't expect miracles of yourself. The key is to make gradual changes that will fit in with your lifestyle and last a lifetime.

It is really important to be patient and have realistic expectations. Think about how long it took to put that weight on. Twelve months? Two years? Don't expect to lose it overnight. There's no magic bullet. Losing body fat is a slow and steady business, but it's much more likely to be permanent.

Moderation is the key. There is no need to avoid any foods totally if you enjoy them—all foods can be included as part of a healthy eating plan. Obviously you need to set some limits, but cutting out all your favourite foods and feeling guilty about eating is not the way to go. Remember, your new eating plan needs to be for life. It means eating right, not necessarily less.

But none of this will work if you don't get moving. It's essential to include some regular physical activity in your day. It's not only important for weight management, it's good for your heart, your bones, for reducing diabetes risk and for managing stress.

5 STEPS TO DEVELOPING GOOD EATING HABITS

1. Listen to your appetite and avoid non-hungry eating—this is the eating you do when bored, stressed or upset. Find alternative ways of coping with these feelings rather than heading for the fridge. You need to find other activities that provide you with the pleasure you get from food—write yourself a list!

2. Focus on what you should eat rather than what you shouldn't—if you fill up on the foods your body needs each day, there won't be much room left for the rest! Eating small amounts often and choosing foods that are satisfying will also help—this is where the GI is important as low GI foods generally keep you fuller for longer.

3. Relax and enjoy your meals, eat slowly and always sit down to eat—you are more likely to be satisfied if you do. Try to avoid eating on the run and get out of the habit of eating while you are doing other things such as watching TV or working.

4. Stock your cupboards with the foods you plan to eat (see pages 132–134 for your healthy low GI shopping list) and avoid buying the foods you want to eat less of. This will be easier if you shop with a list and not when you are hungry!

5. Don't try to change everything overnight or cut out all your favourite foods—this is not sustainable! It is much easier to make one or two changes at a time and to still include a little of what you enjoy.

Don't diet. Focus on eating well and moving more.
Enjoy the foods you eat and make sure you choose
the ones that will give you energy to burn.
And remember, we all need to be active everyday.

Eating well

If you have PCOS, eating well is not just about managing your weight. Eating well can improve your overall health and energy levels, and can help to reduce your risk of heart disease and diabetes. It also means enjoying what you eat. The other thing to remember is that you need to eat in a way that helps to control your insulin levels. This means eating small regular meals and snacks spread across the day and choosing mostly healthy low GI foods. Your healthy low GI eating plan should include the following foods each day:

- fresh vegetables and salads

- fresh fruit

- wholegrain breads and cereals

- low fat dairy products or non-dairy alternatives such as soya

- fish, lean meat, chicken, eggs, legumes and soya products

- small amounts of healthy fats including nuts, seeds, avocado, olives, olive oil, canola oil or peanut oil

We hope you have noticed that we are not asking you to remove a single food group. Cutting out certain sorts of foods is not a long-term solution, nor one which is good for your health or energy levels. Eating the healthy low GI way is about choosing the right foods within *all* the food groups. For most women we see, it simply means swapping one food for another. There's always a tasty substitute. Trust us, we know plenty of them (see page 128).

Remember that when it comes to changing the way we eat, some people find this easy, but for the majority of us, change of any kind is difficult. Unlike altering bad habits such as smoking, changing the food we eat is rarely just a matter of giving up certain foods. A healthy diet contains a wide range of foods, but we need to eat them in the right amounts. The decisions behind what we eat are many and complex, and often some professional advice can help you to make the necessary changes. Helping people improve their diet is what dietitians do every day, so don't be shy. Give a dietitian a call if you need some help to get started. (See 'How to Find a Dietitian' on page 47 to find a dietitian).

WHAT HAPPENS WHEN YOU SEE A DIETITIAN?

Seeing a dietitian is not about being given a list of foods you can't eat or being put on a strict diet. Instead, your dietitian will aim to help you to develop an eating and activity plan to suit your needs and lifestyle and to work with you to set realistic and achievable goals. And these goals are not just about weight—having more energy, improving insulin levels and regulating your periods are just some of the goals you might want to work on with the help of your dietitian. There is no need to worry about being judged by the scales—in fact many dietitians won't weigh you unless this is something that is important to you.

In the UK, dietitians have a minimum of four years of university training and are experts in nutrition and dietetics. They have the knowledge, understanding and clinical training to advise you on the best eating plan to meet your individual needs.

Your first consultation with a dietitian will generally take about an hour and will begin with collecting personal details, weight history, medical history, usual eating patterns and activity levels, and your goals and expectations for your consultations. This information will allow the dietitian to assess your needs and to provide information and education relevant to your situation. The dietitian will then assist you in developing an eating plan to meet your individual needs as well as the information and ideas you need to put this into practice.

The dietitian will generally want to see you again after a few weeks to review your progress and to provide further education as well as answer any questions you may have. How often you see the dietitian will be up to you—some people like to go along every week or two until they achieve their goals, while others only want one or two sessions to obtain the information they need.

To find a dietitian in your area see page 47

How do I change my diet?
Aim to make changes gradually.

Major changes to your diet, for example following a fad diet from a magazine article or current bestseller, are usually short-lived. Identify one aspect of your diet that you want to work on (for example, eating more vegetables) and make that your initial focus.

Attempt the easiest changes first.

Nothing inspires like success, so increase your chances by attacking the easiest changes first. For example, plan to eat one fruit snack each day.

Break big goals into a number of smaller, more achievable goals.

A big goal may be wanting to lose weight. This is unlikely to happen quickly, but it is attainable through gradual, consistent change. Smaller goals could be to exercise for 30 minutes every day and to reduce the saturated-fat content of your diet. Even smaller goals (which are the best way to begin) could be to do a 15 minute walk on alternate days and limit takeaway meals to once a week.

Be prepared for setbacks.

It is normal to experience setbacks when making any type of change and lifestyle changes are no exception. If you find yourself getting off track, don't see this as a failure but as a natural stage in the progression to new habits. Remember, it usually takes about three months for a new change to become a habit. Accept lapses for what they are—you're only human—and get back on track the next day.

> Don't try to change everything overnight—
> start with a few small changes and add more
> as you achieve these.

Moving more with PCOS

Activity and exercise are essential if you want to manage PCOS. It has to be regular and at least some of it has to be aerobic such as walking, cycling or dancing. Regular exercise can help you control your weight, manage your

I was referred to a dietitian by my endocrionologist after being diagnosed with PCOS and insulin resistance. I had a history of heavy, really painful periods, mood swings, bloating, scalp hair loss, difficulties controlling my weight and had been unable to fall pregnant despite trying IVF. At my first meeting I was wearing a size 18–22 and when asked, all I could say was that I wanted to be size 12 again. I had tried so many diets with no long-term success.

The dietitian told me about healthy low GI eating and gave me lots of ideas to improve my current eating habits to reduce fat and incorporate more healthy low GI foods into my meals and snacks. It all sounded very achievable and I was confident that I could fit in a 20–30 minute walk most days. My endocrinologist started me on metformin at this point too.

I saw the dietitian every month and each time I felt I was making positive changes to my diet and gradually increasing my activity levels. I built up to walking an hour most mornings as well as starting a strength training programme at home on alternate days. Most of all I made sure that I ate regularly, including lots of fruit and vegetables, eating more fish and nuts and switching most of my carbohydrate foods to low GI choices. My energy levels improved significantly and after ten months I was a size 14–16! And that was pretty exciting. But even more exciting was the fact that at last I was pregnant! I had a really easy pregnancy—mind you, I stuck carefully to my low GI eating plan and I exercised regularly right up until the birth. The good news was that my blood glucose levels remained well controlled with no signs of gestational diabetes. And as this book was being written, I gave birth to a healthy baby girl.

Lisa, 32

insulin levels and make a real difference to your health and energy levels. Best of all, every little bit counts.

- Exercise and activity speed up your metabolic rate (increasing the amount of energy you use) which helps you to balance your food intake and control your weight.

- Exercise and activity make your muscles more sensitive to insulin, which increases the amount of fat you burn.

A healthy low GI diet has the same effect. Healthy low GI foods reduce the amount of insulin you need, which makes fat easier to burn and harder to store. Since body fat is what you want to get rid of when you lose weight, exercise or activity in combination with a healthy low GI diet makes a lot of sense!

Did you know that research has shown that people who exercise regularly, even if they are overweight or have a family history of diabetes, have significantly less risk of developing diabetes? Exercise also protects against heart disease, with regular exercisers having a much smaller risk of developing cardiovascular disease.

Regular exercise has also been shown to:

- strengthen bones and muscles

- decrease anxiety and depression

- improve general wellbeing and quality of life

- improve blood fats

- reduce blood pressure

- improve strength and flexibility

- reduce body fat and increase lean body mass

- improve physical fitness

- enhance self-esteem and psychological wellbeing

Just a few good reasons to get moving!

What type of exercise and how much?

Ideally you should try to fit in some activity on most days. Research has shown that just 30 minutes of moderate intensity exercise each day can help to improve your health, in particular reducing your risk of heart disease and diabetes. If you prefer, you can break this 30 minutes down to two sessions of 15 minutes or even three sessions of 10 minutes each and you will still see benefits.

If you are trying to lose weight, the more exercise you can do the better. Start with 30 minutes each day and build it up. If you can manage to be active for an hour most days you will certainly see the benefits. If you can't fit this in, do whatever you can—remember every little bit counts!

While aerobic exercise is generally thought of as the most effective for 'fat-burning', and is certainly important, combining aerobic exercise with resistance training will give you even better results. Resistance training (also called strength training or weight training) helps to build muscle and increases your metabolism, assisting with weight loss. Research has also shown the benefits of resistance training for improving insulin resistance, reducing cardiovascular risk factors and improving blood glucose control in people with diabetes.

A balanced exercise programme, including aerobic, resistance and flexibility/stretching exercises will give you the best results. Variety is also important—the body becomes efficient at anything it does repeatedly so after a while you'll stop seeing the results you initially got by doing what you are doing now. This is the time to add something new to your exercise programme!

Our top ten ways to get moving

Exercise doesn't have to mean sweating it out at the gym (unless that's what you like!). The key is to find some activities that you enjoy. If exercise is a chore and you struggle to do it every day it will be too hard to keep up.

There are lots of options when it comes to being more active. Below are 10 ideas to get you moving. You don't have to go solo. Exercising with friends is good for one and all. If you have had an injury of any sort, check it out with your doctor before you start any exercise programme.

Walking

This is one of the best ways to get active as it is easy, you can do it almost anywhere and all you need to get started is a good pair of shoes. You don't have to climb a mountain, and it doesn't have to be a hike or a trek. Simply start the day by walking to work or, if you are not a morning person, try walking home and arrive home stress free! If you don't like walking alone, grab a partner or friend and combine your workout with catching up on the day's news. You could also get off the bus or train a stop or two earlier and walk the rest of the way, or fit in a walk at lunchtime for a chance to stretch and get some fresh air. On the weekend, consider a longer walk in the park or try hiking or mountain climbing.

You could also fit more walking into your day by walking short distances instead of taking the car; walking the kids to school or taking them for a walk to the park; taking the dog for a walk around the block; or catching up with a friend for a walk rather than a coffee.

Dancing

Dancing is a lot of fun as well as being a great way to get your blood pumping. There are a variety of classes available, either through community colleges or privately, including ballroom, ballet, ceroc, funk, jazz, Latin, tango, rock 'n' roll and belly dancing. You don't have to know how—find a beginners class and go along for some fun. Most teachers will tell you that if you can walk you can dance! If you are not brave enough to join a class, or don't have time, clear some room at home, turn your favourite music up loud and start grooving!

Treadmills and exercise bikes

If time is an issue or you are not an outdoors sort of person these are an ideal option. Buy or hire a treadmill or bike for home and you can use it whenever it suits you—without worrying about the weather. You can also save time by combining your exercise with reading (for work or pleasure) or watching your favourite TV show. Otherwise listening to some good music will ensure you keep your heart rate up and will make the time go faster.

Exercise classes

Fitness centres, community colleges and private studios all run a variety of classes such as aerobics, step, boxercise, pump, yoga and pilates. If you are not sure about joining a class, or you can't find one to fit your time schedule, you can buy exercise videos to use at home or try hiring one from your local video shop or library.

Lifting weights

Weight lifting, also known as resistance training or strength training, is something that everyone should be doing on a regular basis. Many women are scared of lifting weights as they think they will 'bulk up', but this is unlikely unless you have a particularly muscly body type and are lifting really heavy weights. What weights can do is help you to become more toned, increase your metabolism, improve your body's sensitivity to insulin and strengthen your bones.

You can use machines or free weights at your local fitness centre where the trainers should be able to help you with a programme. To do it at home all you need to begin is a set of dumbbells and some ankle weights. There are books and videos available to help you or you might want to consider a few sessions with a personal trainer to get you started. One book we would recommend is *Strong Women Stay Young* by Miriam Nelson. Written specifically for women, this book includes an easy to follow strength training programme for home as well as a guide to exercises you can do at the gym.

Play a sport

Netball, basketball, soccer, touch football, tennis or golf to name just a few—why not join your local competition or organise a game with friends?

Swimming and aqua-aerobics

If you like the water, these may be the best exercises for you. Water exercises are also particularly good for anyone with joint problems as your weight is supported in the water. Head to your favourite pool and see what they have to offer. Aqua-aerobic classes are also held at many fitness centres and hospitals.

Rowing

Outdoor or indoor, rowing is a great all-over workout which will have you fit in no time! If you can't see yourself getting out on the water in a rowboat, canoe or kayak, the next best thing is to buy or hire a rowing machine for home or use one at your local fitness centre.

Household chores

Master the art of getting two jobs done at once—your exercise and your household chores. You may not think of these activities as exercise but cleaning, dusting, vacuuming and mopping will all give you a good workout as will washing the car, mowing the lawn, sweeping and digging in the garden. Put on your favourite music while you work and put in your best effort—you won't only get a great workout but you will have the reward of a clean house, shiny car or neat and tidy yard at the end.

A few more ideas . . .

Indoor rock climbing, skiing, ice-skating, skipping, cycling—the possibilities are endless! Pick the activity that you think you will enjoy most and get moving!

Building more activity into your day

In addition to planned exercise, just moving more throughout the day can make a big difference. Cars, computers, dishwashers, washing machines, mobile phones and email mean that many of us get very little activity in our day. Remember, becoming more active means thinking about exercise or movement as an opportunity not an inconvenience. Consider the ways you could get a bit more movement in your day—every little bit counts!

- Take the stairs instead of the lift—make this a policy!

- Wash the car by hand rather than going to the car wash—put the money you save towards a reward for yourself.

- Walk to get the weekend papers rather than getting them delivered—you will feel like you have earned the right to sit in the sun and read when you get back.

- Park a bit further from the shops rather than looking for the closest spot—this will also save the time and frustration of driving around in circles looking for that spot you can never find.

- Walk short distances rather than taking the car—this also saves on petrol and you will be doing your bit for the environment.

Research has shown that we need to take about 7500 steps each day to maintain weight and 10 000 steps to lose weight. If you want to see how much you move (or don't move!), buy a pedometer (step-counter) and see how you go. A pedometer can be a good motivator to moving more. They are available from most sports shops. It's both fun and a challenge. Give it a go! Also, for advice on walking and steps programmes contact www.whi.org.uk.

How to stay motivated? That's not just *your* problem.

Many of the women who talk to us say that they find it difficult to get started with exercise and even more challenging to continue a regular exercise programme. If this sounds like you, you are not alone! Research has shown that of all those who start an exercise programme, only about a third continue with it beyond three months. To increase your chance of success, it is important to think about the things that may help motivate you to start and continue exercising. Here are some pointers which have helped the women we see to get started and to keep going with their exercise programmes:

Women who get active and stay active:

1. Set realistic short-term and long-term goals.

2. Understand the benefits that exercise will provide.

3. Start slowly and gradually increase what they do as it gets easier.

4. Include a variety of activities that are enjoyable and fun.

5. Choose times and locations that are convenient.

6. Make sure their exercise programme is flexible and fits in with their lifestyle.

7. Monitor and reward their progress.

8. Exercise with others—make a commitment to them.

9. Think of exercise as an investment of their time (and a good one at that!) rather than something that takes time.

10. Recognise the rewards exercise is providing, even when the weight isn't dropping off—exercise improves your sensitivity to insulin regardless of weight loss as well as increasing fitness, strength and energy levels.

You can't afford not to exercise!
Find an activity you enjoy and get moving!

PERSONAL TRAINERS

Working with a personal trainer can be a great way to improve your health and fitness. A good trainer will design an exercise programme tailored to your needs and fitness level and provide motivation and support. Many personal trainers now offer services for a reasonable rate and you can choose to use a health club or train at home or outdoors. If cost is an issue, you could train with a group of three or four others with similar fitness levels, or you could just have a few sessions to get you started. If you can, try to budget for at least 10 sessions to help achieve your goals and increase your confidence.

How do I find a good personal trainer?

Many trainers are attached to health clubs, but if you don't belong to one, look in your local newspaper or search online for someone in your area. You can also contact the NRPT (National Register of Personal Trainers) by phone: 0870 200 6010 or via their website: www.nrpt.co.uk. The NRPT will be able to provide the names and contact details of recognised personal trainers in your area. A good trainer should offer you at least one complimentary session to 'try before you buy'. This will ensure that you feel comfortable with them before signing up for ongoing sessions. If you are not sure, try another trainer.

What to expect when you see a personal trainer

In your first session, the trainer will ask you about your current lifestyle and any health or medical problems, as well as your goals and expectations. He or she will then work out a programme to best help you reach those goals. Trainers supervise each of your sessions to make sure you are performing the exercises correctly and to push you to the next step in achieving your goals. They will also help to motivate you when the going gets tough. Remember, though, a trainer can't do the work for you –

it will still be necessary to put in the effort and do some extra exercise outside of your personal training sessions (unless you can afford a trainer every day!)

Discuss payment options with the trainer in your first session. Most will suggest that you sign up for a number of sessions – either weekly or a few times per week, depending on your goals and finances. If you are happy to exercise but just need some guidance on what to do, once a week might be fine, but if you are struggling to get going, you might want to start with a few sessions per week until you build your new habits. If once a week is all you can afford, you could try finding an exercise buddy or buy an exercise video or DVD to help guide and motivate you between your training sessions.

Take care of yourself

Eating well and being active are the cornerstones of managing PCOS, but there are a few other things that you can do to help yourself which are very important for improving your overall health, energy levels and feeling of wellbeing.

Taking care of yourself is essential and what we call the four Ss make up the final part of your four-step plan. This means:

- surviving stress

- sleeping soundly

- seeking support

- stopping smoking

Surviving stress

This really is the S word isn't it? Stress is a part of life for most of us and can't be avoided. While you may be able to eliminate some of the stress in your life, the key to managing stress effectively is to increase your ability to cope with the stresses and strains you face.

The additional problem with stress for women with PCOS is that it can upset hormonal balance, increase blood glucose levels, blood fats and blood pressure, reduce immunity and upset digestion. Stress also sends many of us heading straight for the fridge door!

Unfortunately, PCOS itself tends to create extra stress. First you must you deal with the physical symptoms—excess hair, skin problems, managing weight and, for some, being unable to fall pregnant.

Then there are the emotional consequences of living with PCOS—an often forgotten part of dealing with this condition. Having PCOS can impact significantly on body image and self-esteem and this, in turn, can affect your ability to cope with the problems you face. Enhancing self-esteem and improving body image are an important part of your PCOS management plan.

Remember that it is absolutely normal at some stage to feel fed up, frustrated or overwhelmed by PCOS. At the same time, it is really important to know that it is completely reasonable and understandable to feel like this and it is okay to seek help. If you feel unable to cope on your own you should seek some professional help—find a psychologist or counsellor who can help you to deal with the issues you face.

> My GP referred me to an endocrinologist because I was always tired, gaining weight and had terrible mood swings. After tests it became clear that my routine blood and thyroid function tests were absolutely normal but I had a slight enlargement of the thyroid. We decided to wait

and see . . . and I made an appointment for a follow-up review three months later. By the time the review happened, I had gained 3 kilograms (6½ pounds), and my constant fatigue and mood swings were interfering with my effectiveness as an executive and with my home life.

By this time my endocrinologist suspected PCOS and, on questioning, I realised that my periods were two to three days longer than they had been six months earlier. I also remembered that my hairdresser had commented that the hair on the top of my head was thinning. The endocrinologist also noticed that there was excess hair around my right nipple and naval line. Tests showed that my serum LH was markedly elevated. That's when I was scheduled an internal ultrasound, which showed unequivocal evidence of PCOS. I was prescribed metformin, a healthy low GI diet and aerobic exercise. I lost around 15 kilograms (33 pounds) over a three-month period and started to feel much better about myself—I was even promoted at work!

That's when I decided to do an MBA part-time to further my career, but it all became too much. I found it hard to meet all my deadlines and look after myself properly; I was always rushing. I was too busy to exercise, I ate whatever I could lay my hands on and, worst of all, I forgot to renew my prescription for metformin. It was also a very anxious time for the whole family as my mother was diagnosed with Alzheimer's.

I missed two appointments at the clinic and when I finally went back and jumped on the scales I had put on 17 kilograms (37 pounds). By this time my periods were irregular and I had dark coarse facial hair and acne. I went back on my programme of healthy low GI eating, exercise and metformin. It wasn't easy, but I did get my MBA!

Christine, 28

How Do You Cope with Stress?

	ALWAYS	SOMETIMES	NEVER
Do you exercise regularly?			
Do you communicate feelings to others?			
Do you take time out for activities you enjoy?			
Do you remain positive and optimistic, even during difficult times?			
Do you practise any formal relaxation techniques such as meditation?			
Do you manage your time effectively and get all your important tasks done each day?			

Mostly 'Always'

Congratulations—you should be able to cope well with the stress that life presents you. Managing stress has many important health benefits so keep up the good work!

Mostly 'Sometimes'

You are halfway there but there is more you could be doing to cope with stress. Pick the areas you are not doing so well in and build in some strategies to help. For example, if you are stressed by your never-ending 'to do pile' and never seem to have time for yourself, start with learning to manage your time more effectively—write lists, prioritise and schedule some relaxation time for yourself.

Mostly 'Never'

It is likely that you are not coping well with the stress in your life and this could be impacting negatively on your health and wellbeing. There are many things you could do to increase your ability to deal with stress: starting a regular exercise programme; taking some time out for activities you enjoy; and finding someone to talk to about your feelings would be a great start.

Thousands of people tend to turn to food when under pressure. If you are like them you need to find other ways of coping. It may seem a bit like homework, but it is useful to write yourself a list of all those things you would like to do that you never get time to fit in—most of us have lots of these! This list can be a useful prompt, especially if you stick it on the fridge door!

Here are some ideas that many women with PCOS have told us that they find useful. These suggestions may help to get you started, but don't forget to add your own:

Read a good book	Have a bubble bath
Spend time in the garden	Write to a friend
Clean out your wardrobe	Have a massage
Go to bed early and read	Sit in the sun and read the
Redecorate your house	paper
Listen to music	Watch a good movie
Give yourself a pedicure	Buy yourself some flowers
Have a haircut	Have a weekend away
Visit the zoo	Learn something new
Have a facial	Look at photographs
Go for a drive	Buy some new clothes

You may wonder if managing your stress levels is really that important—we would like to *stress* that it is! Numerous studies have demonstrated the links between chronic stress and poor health including a greater risk of cardiovascular disease and reduced immune function. And a recent study

SLEEP DISTURBANCE

It's not uncommon for women with PCOS to have difficulties sleeping, such as having trouble getting off to sleep or experiencing disrupted sleep. This may be due to hormonal fluctuations, particularly around the time of your periods, and may also be a result of stress. Carrying extra weight, particularly around the middle, can also lead to sleep disturbances including sleep apnoea. This is a condition where breathing is disrupted during sleep due to blockages to the windpipe—symptoms include snoring and stopping breathing for short periods while asleep. If you suffer from any form of sleep disturbance on an ongoing basis you should seek professional help. Poor sleep can lead to excessive daytime sleepiness and will reduce energy levels, increase stress and make exercise more difficult.

looking at the effects of stress on cellular ageing found that healthy premenopausal women with the highest stress levels had markers of biological ageing which were equivalent to at least one decade of additional ageing compared to the low stressed women. This should be enough to make everyone seriously consider how to reduce their stress levels!

In our experience, many of the women who do not respond well with diet, exercise and metformin are those who are under a significant amount of stress. And managing this stress usually leads to success.

So if you don't already, we encourage you to consider that stress management is just as important as other parts of your PCOS management plan such as diet, exercise and medication. Work out what causes your stress and develop a stress management plan. Different things work for different people so work out the best plan of action for you. This might mean scheduling some time-out, booking in for a regular massage, taking up meditation or seeing a psychologist to talk through the issues you are dealing with. Do whatever it takes to reduce your stress levels—your health depends on it!

Sleeping soundly

Getting enough sleep is vital. A lack of sleep can have many negative consequences—reducing immunity, increasing the level of stress hormones and worsening insulin resistance. In fact a number of studies in healthy subjects have shown that sleep deprivation leads to a significant worsening of insulin sensitivity, even over short periods of time. Being tired also worsens memory, reduces productivity and makes it harder to get enthusiastic about exercising and eating well. Finally, lack of sleep can make it harder to cope with stress.

If you're not getting enough sleep, you're not alone. While most adults need at least eight hours sleep, statistics show that a large proportion of the population sleep for seven hours or less each night. Most adults also report difficulties sleeping at some time.

Our message to you is that sleep is just as important as diet and exercise. Make an effort to get your eight hours and if you have difficulties sleeping, try the tips below or seek some professional help.

Tips for getting a good night's sleep:

- Exercise regularly but avoid strenuous exercise close to bedtime.

- Go to bed and get up at the same time each day (+/- an hour on Sunday!).

- Relax for an hour before bed—avoid stimulating activities such as scary movies and loud music.

- Try not to work right up to bedtime and make sure you finish your work day by writing down a list of things you need to do tomorrow so that your brain doesn't work hard to remember them all night.

- Make sure your bedroom is quiet, dark and a comfortable temperature before your go to bed—noise, light and being too hot or cold will all make it harder to get a good night's sleep.

- If you have trouble getting off to sleep, get up and read for 20 minutes, try a glass of warm milk or listen to a relaxation tape. Research has shown that they do work.

- Lavender essential oil has been shown to help with sleep—try burning some in an oil burner or sprinkle a few drops on your pillow.

Seeking support

Having a good support team can make all the difference when you have PCOS. Many of the women we see comment on the fact that they feel very much alone in living with their condition and feel that no one else understands what they are going through. Talking about these feelings and meeting other women in the same boat can be a big help.

The good news is that there *is* support out there for women with PCOS. From formal PCOS support groups to understanding health professionals you can find the care and attention that you need.

Your team of health professionals might include a GP, endocrinologist, gynaecologist and dietitian. You may also want to seek the help of a psychologist, exercise physiologist or personal trainer and natural health practitioner. PCOS

ABOUT PCOS SUPPORT GROUPS

PCOS support groups provide information, education and support to women with PCOS as well as their partners, family and friends. From face-to-face meetings and email chat groups to newsletters and websites, they provide the opportunity for women to come together for mutual support and friendship and provide the information to empower women with PCOS to take charge of their condition. Many of these groups also work hard to raise the public awareness of PCOS and the effects it has on the lives of so many women, and encourage research which could lead to a cure or more effective treatment. The details for support groups are included in the back of this book—we encourage you to contact them and find out how you can get involved.

support groups can provide you with valuable information and contact with others through meetings, newsletters, websites and email discussion groups.

You could also seek out other groups such as infertility support groups. Ask your health professional for a referral or look in the *Yellow Pages* for contact details.

Stopping smoking

If you smoke, giving up smoking is one of the most important things you can do to improve your health and the health of those around you. Everyone these days is well aware that smoking increases the risk of heart disease and cancer. Did you also know that smoking worsens insulin sensitivity and reduces fertility? All smokers with PCOS should quit and this is particularly important if you are trying to fall pregnant.

Quitting smoking is not easy, so if you have made the

decision to quit but need some help in doing so, talk to your local doctor or visit the website: www.smokenders.com

Take time out to take care of yourself.
Reducing and managing stress and getting
enough sleep will give you the time and energy
to focus on making other lifestyle changes.
Seek support if you need to.
If you are a smoker stop now!

CHAPTER 4

PUTTING THE GI TO WORK IN YOUR DAY

I understand GI but what is GL and what does it mean?
The optimum diet for women with PCOS
Seven dietary guidelines for women with PCOS
The flavour on fluids
A quick guide to healthy low GI eating
Putting it all together—a typical day the low GI way
Eating out
Your healthy low GI shopping list
Your low GI menus

This chapter lays out the practical part of *The New Glucose Revolution* and explains how to make the change to the healthy low GI way of eating.

Remember that eating the healthy low GI way is not a diet. It means changing your eating habits in a way that will last you a lifetime. It's not about weighing, counting or measuring and it's not about eating foods you dislike or cutting out the foods you enjoy most. What it is about is eating the right foods—the foods that fill you up, give you more energy and improve your health and, best of all, your PCOS symptoms.

There are plenty of choices when it comes to healthy low GI eating which is why the women we see comment that this is the easiest 'diet' they have ever followed. They don't feel hungry; they can still eat foods they enjoy; they have more energy and their cravings subside. In essence, they feel good and their new way of eating feels sustainable. And if it's sustainable it's likely to work.

I understand GI but what is GL and what does it mean?

It is important to consider both the GI of the food and the amount of carbohydrate it contains, i.e. the total glycaemic load—this is a rough measure of the effect of your meal or snack on your blood glucose and insulin levels. You can calculate the glycaemic load (GL) by multiplying the GI by the amount of carbohydrate per serve and then dividing by 100. For example, 1 cup of watermelon has a GI of 72 and a carbohydrate content of 10 g, giving a GL of 7, while a medium apple has a GI of 38 and a carbohydrate content of 15 g, giving a GL of 6. So although watermelon has a higher GI than other fruits, its high water content means that eaten in moderate amounts, it is comparable

LOW GI OR LOW CARB?

When you have PCOS, reducing insulin levels is important. When it comes to the food you eat, the key to reducing insulin levels is reducing the glycaemic load (GL) of your diet. There are two ways to do this—reduce the GI of your diet overall or reduce your carbohydrate intake. Many of the women we see try the second option first because it sounds easy to cut carbohydrate foods out of their diet. While this may help short term, it is not the answer for long-term good health and management of your PCOS.

The reason for this is that low carbohydrate diets can worsen insulin resistance and they eliminate many of the foods we know are important for good health and reducing risk of diseases such as cancer, heart disease and type 2 diabetes. Low carbohydrate diets also tend to lower energy levels, making exercise more difficult. A diet based on low GI foods, on the other hand, gives you the best of both worlds—enough carbohydrate for optimum insulin sensitivity, nutrition and energy levels without an excessive GL.

If weight loss is a goal, high carbohydrate diets are probably not the answer for you either—as with most things, moderation is the key. Whether you have a high or moderate carbohydrate intake, however, you should choose mostly healthy low GI carbs.

The good news is that eating the low GI way will mean that you feel fuller and will be less likely to overeat. This means that measuring, counting and weighing your food can be a thing of the past. You will also find that when you are choosy about your carbohydrate, your insulin levels will be lower and you will therefore burn more fat. Over time, and combined with some regular exercise, this will result in weight loss.

to other fruits with a lower GI. GL tells us that small amounts of a high GI food are unlikely to have a big impact on blood glucose and insulin levels while large serves of a low GI food can still raise blood glucose and insulin levels significantly. Portion size does matter! However, because low GI foods are more satisfying, we recommend you choose foods mostly on the basis of GI, not GL.

The optimum diet for women with PCOS

The optimum diet for women with PCOS is one that is low in saturated fat and contains moderate amounts of protein and carbohydrate, with most of the carbohydrate choices being low GI. It should contain plenty of vegetables, salads, fruit, legumes and wholegrains.

This type of eating plan will help achieve weight management, boost energy levels, improve insulin sensitivity and reduce the risk of health problems such as diabetes and heart disease.

To make it easy for you we have developed seven dietary guidelines. These aren't rules, they are a simple guide to inspire you to improve your eating habits for life. Then, to help you to implement these guidelines we explain in detail how you can translate them into daily meals and snacks. Finally we finish this section with a shopping list and sample meal plans to get you started.

I have asthma and over a very wheezy six-month period I had to have two back-to-back courses of high-dose steroids by mouth (as well as antibiotics). That's when I put on 10 kilograms (22 pounds) predominantly around my middle and upper thighs. Despite working out in the gym doing aerobic exercises 3–4 times a week and going on what I thought was a weight-reducing diet I was absolutely unable to shed any of the weight I had put on during the steroid treatment. So I went to see my doctor who sent me off to an endocrinologist. All the tests he did seemed absolutely normal. However, he did say that I might be insulin resistant and recommended a healthy low GI diet which I followed religiously—and in the first ten days lost 2.5 kilograms (5½ pounds). It's such an easy diet to follow, I recommended it to many of my friends and to my daughter.
Didi, 56

Seven dietary guidelines for women with PCOS

1. Eat seven or more servings of vegetables and fruit each day.

2. Choose wholegrain breads and cereals with a low GI.

3. Eat more legumes (dried beans, peas and lentils).

4. Include nuts in your diet regularly.

5. Eat more fish and seafood, particularly oily fish like salmon and sardines.

6. Choose lean meats and low fat dairy products.

7. Choose monounsaturated and omega-3 polyunsaturated fats such as olive and canola oil, fish, nuts, seeds and avocado.

1. Eat seven or more servings of vegetables and fruit every day

Fruit and vegetables should form a major part of any healthy eating plan. They are rich sources of vitamins, minerals, antioxidants and phytochemicals, all of which are important for good health and can help to protect you against diseases such as cancer and cardiovascular disease. They are also high in fibre, helping to fill you up and, apart from avocado and olives which contain 'healthy' monounsaturated fats, fruits and vegetables are very low in fat.

Apart from the starchy vegetables: potato, sweet potato, corn, taro and yam, most vegetables have very little carbohydrate so do not have a GI value. Potatoes generally have a high GI, while sweet potato, corn, taro and yam have a relatively low GI. This means that if you are a big potato eater, you should try to replace some potato for these lower GI starchy vegetables. And when you do choose potato, try to go for the baby new potatoes, which have a lower GI than other varieties. Vegetables like pumpkin and carrot have a GI value but there is very little carbohydrate in a normal serve of these vegetables so we suggest that you consider them as 'free foods'. All green vegetables and salad vegetables can also be eaten freely and you should aim to eat at least five serves of vegetables each day— one serve is half a cup of cooked vegetables or one cup of salad vegetables.

When choosing vegetables, variety is the key—don't just stick with the same old varieties like beans, carrots and peas. Spinach, bok choy, broccoli, cauliflower, cabbage, brussels sprouts, pepper, tomato, cucumber, rocket, asparagus, courgette, mangetout, and aubergine—the possibilities are endless. Why not buy something different each time you shop? Aim to make your plate as colourful as possible. Ask your greengrocer what's in season right now.

All fruits contain carbohydrate from their natural sugar content. Most fruits have a low or moderate GI, with the exception of watermelon, which has a high GI. This doesn't mean you need to avoid higher GI fruits like melons—these fruits have a lower carbohydrate intake due to the amount of water they contain so their GL, or overall effect on blood glucose and insulin levels, is still relatively small. In general, temperate fruits like apples and pears tend to have a lower GI and tropical fruits like melons and pineapple tend to have a moderate to high GI. Try to include a variety of fruit as part of your low GI eating plan and aim for at least two serves each day—one serve is a medium piece like an apple or banana or 2–3 smaller pieces like plums and apricots.

Use the following ideas to get your seven serves each day:

Breakfast

- Include fruit (fresh, canned in natural juice or dried) with your breakfast cereal.

- Try a fresh fruit smoothie for a quick but satisfying breakfast meal.

- For a more substantial breakfast, add some vegetables on your toast—try asparagus, mushrooms, tomato and onion or sliced tomato and avocado.

- Mushrooms, asparagus and tomato are also good added to omelettes.

Lunch

- Add plenty of salad vegetables on your sandwich—try tomato, lettuce, cucumber, sprouts, beetroot, grated carrot and pepper.

- For toasted sandwiches go for tomato, pepper, mushroom, sweet potato, olives, courgette and aubergine.

- Use avocado as a spread on your sandwich instead of butter.

- Salads are a great way to fill up at lunchtime and the possibilities are endless—don't stick with lettuce, tomato and cucumber, try adding mangetout, red or green pepper, corn, green beans, steamed broccoli, asparagus, roasted sweet potato and aubergine, sundried tomatoes and a few cubes of avocado or some olives.

- For colder weather soups are a great way to get more vegetables into your diet—try pumpkin, sweet potato, lentil, split pea, minestrone or tomato.

Dinner

- Include vegetables or salads with all main meals—serve them steamed, seasoned with fresh or dried herbs, or with a dressing made from olive oil, lemon juice, balsamic vinegar and garlic.

- Always have some frozen vegetables handy for when you haven't had time to shop for fresh varieties.

- If you don't like vegetables on their own, add them to stir-fries, curries, casseroles and grated into mince.

- Choose vegetable-based dishes when eating out or ask for a side salad with your meal.

Snacks and Desserts

- Fruit and grated vegetables such as carrot and courgette can be added into cakes and muffins.

- Choose fruit for snacks—fruit is widely available, inexpensive and easy to eat, without the added fat and sugar found in many other snack foods.

- Serve raw vegetables such as celery, carrot, cucumber, red or green pepper, broccoli or cauliflower florets as a snack served with a low fat dip or salsa.

- Make fruit the basis of your desserts—try baked apples, fruit crumbles, filo with fruit, and tinned fruit with low fat custard, yoghurt or ice-cream.

2. Eat wholegrain breads and cereals with a low glycaemic index

Cereal grains including rice, wheat, oats, barley, rye and products made from them (including bread, pasta, breakfast cereal and flours) are the most concentrated sources of carbohydrate that we eat, so have a major impact on the GI of our diet.

Wholegrain breads and cereals have many health benefits. Most have a lower glycaemic index than refined cereal grains and they are also nutritionally superior, containing higher levels of fibre, vitamins, minerals and phytochemicals. We know from studies that higher consumption of cereal fibre and wholegrains is associated with a reduced incidence of type 2 diabetes, cancer and heart disease.

Unfortunately, our Western diet tends to be based on highly processed grains and flours, which are quickly digested and result in a much greater rise in blood glucose and insulin levels than is desirable. Since high insulin levels are something you want to avoid when you have PCOS, substituting processed grains and cereals for those with a lower GI is a very important part of making the change to a healthy low GI diet. Lower GI choices include oats, wholegrain and sourdough breads, bulgur, barley, quinoa, most types of pasta and noodles, and longer grain varieties of rice such as basmati.

To eat more breads and cereals with a low GI try the following ideas:

Breakfast

- Porridge is one of the best breakfast choices around— it is inexpensive, has no added fats or sugars and is really satisfying, particularly on a cold morning! Add some stewed apple, a few sultanas and a sprinkle of cinnamon for sweetness and top with low fat milk or soya milk. Remember to choose the whole oats rather than the instant varieties, which have a much higher GI due to all that processing.

- In warmer weather choose cereals based on wheat bran, psyllium and oats such as natural muesli and All-Bran™.

- For those who prefer toast, choose granary, pumpernickel or sourdough bread or try a granary roll.

Lunch

- For sandwiches, go for grainy breads made with barley, rye, linseed, triticale, sunflower seed, oats, soya and cracked wheat. You could also try sourdough or pumpernickel breads.

- Barley can be added to soups to make a satisfying winter lunch.

- Pita bread also has a lower GI—try a pita filled with hommous and tabbouli (made from cracked wheat) or for colder weather a pita pizza topped with tomato, peppers, mushrooms, avocado, a few olives and a sprinkle of grated cheese.

- If you are buying lunch out, try a small pasta with tomato based sauce, Asian noodle soups or tandoori chicken with basmati rice.

Dinner

- Choose Asian noodles, rice or egg noodles in place of rice.

- Try medium GI rice such as basmati.

- Barley can be added into soups and casseroles or used in place of rice—it has a nutty, chewy texture.

Snacks and Desserts

- Wholegrain fruit loaf with ricotta makes a satisfying snack for those with a sweet tooth.

- Baked pita bread is a healthy alternative to chips, served with salsa or hommous.

- Try wholegrain crispbreads topped with ricotta, avocado or hommous and sliced tomato.

- For dessert you could try a fruit crumble with oat topping, creamed rice made with medium GI rice, or bread and butter pudding made with wholegrain fruit loaf.

3. Eat more legumes (beans, peas and lentils)

For a low GI food that's easy on the budget, versatile, filling, low in kilojoules and nutritious, look no further than legumes—that bag of dried kidney beans, or packet of lentils or can of chickpeas in the kitchen cupboard! Whether you buy dried beans and cook them yourself at home, or opt for the very convenient, time-saving canned varieties, you are choosing one of nature's lowest GI foods.

Legumes are also high in fibre—both soluble and insoluble—and packed with nutrients providing a valuable source of protein, carbohydrate, B vitamins, folate and minerals. Sprouted dried beans—such as mung, soya, chickpeas and lentils—are excellent sources of vitamin C and are great eaten raw in a salad or stir-fried. Legumes are an important part of the healthy low GI way of eating. Try and put them on the menu at least twice a week, more often if you are vegetarian.

So, what are legumes? Legumes (also known as pulses) are the edible dried seeds found inside the mature pods of legumious plants (e.g. beans, peas and lentils). Nutritionally, they are quite different from fresh, young green beans and peas which don't have as much protein or fibre because their water content is high.

Legumes can be bought either dried or canned. Canned legumes are ready to use (they only need heating through) and meals based on these are much faster to prepare than meat-based meals. Dried legumes need a little more pre-paration—most need to be soaked before cooking—but are worth the effort and can be frozen in small batches so they are ready to use at any time. Soaked or cooked beans can be kept in an airtight container for several days in the fridge. All legumes have a low GI, including dried and canned varieties, although the canned varieties are a little higher than those you cook yourself.

Thanks to a tendency to cause intestinal gas, legumes have generally had a bad name. But not all legumes will make you windy, and not everyone has the problem. Cooking legumes thoroughly in fresh water (not in the water you soaked them in) and rinsing the canned varieties helps; as does eating them regularly—it can improve your tolerance.

Tofu (soya bean curd) is an easy way of using soya. It has a mild flavour itself but absorbs the flavours of other foods, making it delicious when it's been marinated in soya sauce, ginger and garlic and tossed into a stir-fry. Tofu contains very little carbohydrate so doesn't have a GI value.

With such variety and versatility, incorporating legumes into your meals a few times a week is easy—here are some ideas to help you to make these 'superfoods' a more regular part of your diet.

Breakfast

- Baked beans on toast make a easy and satisfying breakfast.

- Try scrambling silken tofu in place of eggs—add some fresh or dried herbs and chopped tomato and sauté in a little olive oil.

Lunch

- Lentil, split pea or minestrone soup all make a satisfying winter lunch.

- Baked bean toasted sandwiches—an easy all-time favourite!

- Add a can of three bean mix or some chickpeas to create a salad that really fills you up.

- Lentils or chickpeas can be made into burgers and served on a roll or pita bread. If you don't have time to make your own burgers, pre-prepared varieties can be found in the chilled section of the supermarket. A great alternative for the barbecue.

- Spread hommous (made from chickpeas) on your sandwich in place of butter.

Dinner

- Add red kidney beans to mince to serve with tacos, burritos, pasta or rice.

- Chickpeas have a nutty flavour and go well in curries and stir-fries.

- Make some dahl (lentils cooked with spices) as an accompaniment to your next curry.

- Green soya beans make a tasty addition to a stir-fry— they have a nutty texture and can be bought frozen in most Asian grocery stores.

- Add cannellini, borlotti or black eye beans to stews and casseroles.

- Firm tofu can be cubed, marinated and added into stir-fries or threaded onto skewers with vegetables to make kebabs for the barbecue or grill.

- Substitute lentils in place of mince in dishes such as cottage pie and lasagne.

Snacks and Desserts

- Silken tofu can be used in place of cream cheese to make desserts such as cheesecake.

- Roasted chickpeas or soya beans make a tasty and satisfying snack.

- Try a small tin of baked beans or four bean mix for a snack if you are really hungry.

- For a healthy dip go for hommous or puree bean spread with carrot and celery sticks.

COOKING WITH BEANS AND PULSES

Dried legumes: dried beans and peas need soaking and cooking before you use them in your meals. Lentils and split peas cook much faster and don't need soaking.

- To *soak* beans, place them in a saucepan and cover with two to three times their volume of cold water—soak overnight or during the day. If time is limited, take a shortcut by adding three times the volume of water to rinsed beans, bringing to a boil for a few minutes then removing from heat and letting them soak for an hour.

- To *cook*, drain off the soaking water, add fresh water, and bring to a boil then simmer until beans are tender. Use the directions on the packet as a time guide.

- Don't add salt to the cooking water—it slows down water absorption so cooking takes longer.

- Don't cook beans in the water they have soaked in. Substances that contribute to flatulence are leached from the beans into the soaking and cooking waters.

Canned legumes: most legumes are available canned, making cooking with beans quick and easy. One 400 g can of beans substitutes for ¾ cup of dried beans.

---

4. Include nuts regularly in your diet

Nuts are a food that most people enjoy but few people eat regularly, particularly if they are watching their weight. The good news is that a number of large studies have now shown a relationship between regular nut consumption and a reduced risk of both heart disease and type 2 diabetes. Eaten in small amounts nuts have also been shown to assist with weight control as they are satisfying and therefore stop you snacking on other foods.

Nuts are a healthy choice because they contain:

- very little saturated fat (the fats are predominantly mono- or polyunsaturated)

- dietary fibre

- vitamin E, an antioxidant believed to help prevent heart disease

- folate, copper and magnesium, nutrients thought to protect against heart disease

Walnuts and pecans also contain some omega-3 fats, while linseeds are very rich in omega-3s, lignans and plant estrogens. When freshly ground, linseeds have a subtle nutty flavour and make a great addition to breads, muffins, biscuits and cereals.

Remember to choose the unsalted variety—salted nuts are usually roasted in saturated fat. And stick to a handful a day if you are watching your weight.

Some easy ways to eat more nuts include:

Breakfast

- Sprinkle a mixture of nuts and seeds over your cereal.

- Use a spread such as peanut, almond or cashew butter on your toast in place of butter or margarine.

Lunch

- Add a handful of walnuts or pine nuts to your salad.

- Tahini (sesame seed paste) can be used as a spread on sandwiches or in salads in place of mayonnaise.

Dinner

- Add nuts and seeds to your favourite meals—try peanuts or sesame seeds in a stir-fry, cashews with a curry, or crushed macadamias with fish or chicken.

- Pesto (ground pine nuts, basil, garlic and olive oil) makes a good pasta sauce or accompaniment to meat or fish.

- Tahini can be used as an alternative to sour cream on potatoes or drizzled over roasted vegetables.

Snacks and Desserts

- Enjoy nuts as a snack. Although high in fat, nuts make a healthy substitute for less nutritious high fat snacks such as potato crisps, chocolate and biscuits. Just be careful not to eat too many—limit to one handful (about 30 grams) each day!

- Wholegrain crackers or toast with nut spread make a satisfying snack.

- Nuts and seeds can be added to baked goods—try walnuts, hazelnuts and almond meal in cakes and muffins; and sunflower seeds, sesame seeds and linseeds in bread.

5. Eat more fish and seafood

Fish, particularly oily fish, are the best source of long chain omega-3 fatty acids, fats which offer valuable health benefits. These types of fats can help to reduce blood clotting and inflammatory reactions and studies have shown that regular fish consumption is linked to a reduced risk of coronary heart disease. In fact, just one serving of fish a week may reduce the risk of a fatal heart attack by 40 per cent. Our bodies only make small amounts of these fatty acids and so we rely on dietary sources, especially fish and seafood, for them. You should try to eat fish at least twice a week.

Fresh fish that contain the highest amounts of omega-3 fats include:

- swordfish

- atlantic salmon

- southern bluefin tuna

- silver perch

- atlantic, pacific and spanish mackerel (blue mackerel)

Canned fish can also provide omega-3 fats, good sources being:

- mackerel

- salmon

- sardines

Try to choose varieties canned in springwater where possible. If you choose fish canned in oil, go for those in olive or canola oil.

You could easily include fish in your diet at least twice a week by having one main meal of fresh fish and a serving of canned salmon or sardines for lunch or breakfast at least once a week.

Just remember not to cook your fish in solid (saturated)

A WORD ABOUT FISH AND MERCURY

While there are many benefits of eating fish, if you are pregnant you do need to be careful about the types of fish you eat. Some fish contain high levels of mercury which can be harmful to your baby.

FSA (Food Standards Agency United Kingdom) recently revised their guidelines on mercury in fish. They advise that pregnant women, women planning pregnancy and young children can continue to consume a variety of fish as part of a healthy diet but should limit their consumption of certain species. Shark (flake), marlin and swordfish should be consumed no more than once per fortnight with no other fish to be consumed during that fortnight. For orange roughy (also sold as sea perch) and catfish, their advice is to consume no more than one serve per week, with no other fish being consumed during that week. Most other varieties of fish caught and sold in the UK contain low levels of mercury and can be eaten without concern.

For more information on the subject consult the website www.food.gov.uk

fat. That means avoiding eating fried fish from fast-food restaurants, even if they say cooked in 'vegetable oil'. If you eat pre-cooked breaded (crumbed) frozen-fish products choose low fat varieties or those that have been cooked in canola oil. You can now get frozen fish products without the crumbs and these would make an even better choice.

If you don't eat fish or seafood you can also get some omega-3 fatty acids from plant foods. Good sources include linseed, canola, walnut and soyabean oils. There are also small amounts in walnuts, linseeds, pecans, soyabeans, baked beans, wheat germ and green leafy vegetables.

To increase your intake of fish, try the following ideas:

Breakfast

- Sardines on toast will fill you up in the morning and give you a good dose of omega-3s.

- Try an omelette with smoked salmon.

Lunch

- Add tuna or salmon to a sandwich or salad.

- For something different, try salmon or tuna rissoles on a roll with lettuce and avocado.

- Grilled fish with salad makes a healthy lunch choice if eating out.

Dinner

- Home-made fish and chips is a quick and easy meal to prepare—wrap fish in foil with lemon juice and herbs and bake in the oven along with sweet potato chips (slice and brush with olive oil—bake on tray in oven). Serve with salad or steamed vegetables.

- Try adding tuna or salmon to pasta with a tomato sauce and some vegetables.

- Barbecue fish makes a healthy alternative to sausages and fatty meats.

6. Eat lean meats and low fat dairy foods

Scientists have known for years that a diet high in saturated fat raises cholesterol levels and increases heart disease risk. More recently, research has also implicated these fats in both insulin resistance and obesity—we burn saturated fat poorly compared to other fats, so it tends to be stored as body fat more readily. In contrast, our bodies are more likely to use omega-3 polyunsaturated fatty acids (PUFAs) and monounsaturated fatty acids (MUFAs) for energy rather than storage.

Reducing your intake of saturated fat doesn't mean that you need to avoid red meat and dairy products. They are good sources of protein, iron and calcium, so as long as you choose lean cuts of meat and low fat dairy products you can still include these foods in moderation as part of a healthy diet.

If you enjoy meat, we suggest eating lean red meat two or three times a week, and accompanying it with salad and vegetables. Trim all visible fat from meat and remove the skin (and the fat just below it) from chicken. Game meats such as rabbit and venison are not only lean but are also good sources of omega-3 fatty acids, as are organ meats such as liver and kidney. If you choose not to eat red meat or are trying to reduce your intake, legumes and tofu are a good alternative as they can provide the protein, iron and zinc that is also found in red meat.

Quorn™ products are another healthy vegetarian option, made from a mushroom species 'mycoprotein'. It is nutritious and contains high-quality protein and fibre. It is also low in total fat and saturated fat.

Replacing full fat dairy foods with reduced fat, low fat or fat free varieties will also help you reduce your saturated fat intake. Dairy products including milk, yoghurt and cheese are among the richest sources of calcium in our diet. They also provide protein, and a number of important vitamins and minerals including vitamin B12, phosphorus, magnesium and zinc.

Alternatively you could choose calcium-fortified soya products such as soya milk and soya yoghurt. Soya products contain mostly polyunsaturated fat and the protein in soya

PHYTOESTROGENS: PROTECTION FROM PLANTS

Phytoestrogens are natural plant chemicals found in foods such as fruit, vegetables, nuts and soya foods. Research shows that people who consume high levels of phytoestrogens enjoy better health and live longer. Phytoestrogens can help to reduce the symptoms of menopause and can lower cholesterol levels and protect against cancer. You can increase your intake of phytoestrogens by eating legumes, tofu and nuts regularly, switching from dairy to soya milk and eating breads and cereals containing soya and linseed.

products can help to lower cholesterol levels. Soya products are also a source of omega-3 fatty acids and phytoestrogens. When purchasing soya products, check labels for total fat content of no more than 3–5%.

Much of the saturated fat we consume these days comes from pre-prepared packaged and takeaway foods; in fact, most fast-food restaurants cook with saturated fat (from either animal or vegetable sources). Until these restaurants make an effort to reduce the saturated fat content of their products, it's best to eat as little fried fast food as possible.

We used to think that eating high cholesterol foods such as eggs, shrimp and other shellfish would raise our blood cholesterol levels. We now know that our liver compensates for the increased cholesterol intake by reducing cholesterol production, although a small percentage of people have an inherited condition called familial hypercholesterolemia, which impairs this self-regulation. This means that most people could eat an egg a day, for example, without harming their heart.

To enhance your intake of omega-3 fats we suggest that you eat omega-3 enriched eggs (if you can find them), which have about six times more ALA and DHA than regular eggs. These enriched eggs are produced by feeding the hens a diet that is naturally rich in omega-3s (including canola and linseeds).

You can include lean meats and low fat dairy products in your diet in the following ways:

Breakfast

- Try poached or scrambled eggs on toast or an omelette.

- Fruit smoothies make a great breakfast when you are on the go and you don't have time to make your own.

- Low fat yoghurt is a tasty accompaniment to muesli.

Lunch

- Sandwiches or rolls can be filled with chicken and avocado, lean roast beef and mustard, turkey and cranberry, sliced lamb with hommous, egg and lettuce, or lean ham and salad.

- If you prefer toasted sandwiches try chicken and avocado, ham, cheese and tomato or ricotta, sundried tomato and rocket.

- Dress up your salad with lean roast meat, sliced chicken breast, a boiled egg or some cubes of low fat feta cheese.

- Frittata made with eggs, low fat milk, chopped vegetables, lean ham, fresh herbs and low fat cheese makes a tasty weekend lunch or brunch served with salad.

- Soups are a great winter warmer—try chicken and sweetcorn, beef and vegetable, or lamb shank and barley.

- For a variation on your usual sandwich, try a pita bread filled with hommous, tabbouli and sliced chicken breast or roast lamb.

Dinner

- Go for lean meats—marinated and grilled, or pan-fried with a little olive or canola oil.

- Beef and chicken can be sliced into strips and stir-fried with vegetables.

- For the barbecue choose lean steak, marinated chicken breast or kebabs.

- Use lean meats in curries and casseroles and, if you have time, cook the day before, refrigerate and skim fat from top the next day before reheating to serve.

- Low fat yoghurt and ricotta mixed with chives makes a low fat alternative to sour cream on vegetables or Mexican food.

Snacks and Desserts

- Fruit smoothies or low fat milkshakes make a satisfying calcium-packed snack.

- Yoghurt is always a quick and easy option.

- Try a glass of low fat hot chocolate to satisfy those chocolate cravings.

- Low fat flavoured milk or soya milk make a good snack on the run.

- Ricotta can be used as topping for crackers or spread on fruit loaf.

WHY DO I NEVER SEE A GI VALUE FOR MEAT OR CHEESE?

The foods we eat contain three main nutrients—protein, carbohydrate and fat. Some foods, such as meat, are high in protein, while bread is high in carbohydrate and butter is high in fat. It is necessary for us to consume a variety of foods (in varying proportions) to provide all three nutrients, but the GI applies only to foods containing carbohydrate. It is impossible for us to measure a GI value for foods which contain negligible carbohydrate. These foods include meat, fish, chicken, eggs, cheese, nuts, oils, cream, butter and most vegetables. There are other nutritional aspects which you could consider in choosing these foods, for example the amount and type of fats they contain.

- Add a spoonful of low fat custard, frozen yoghurt or ice-cream to fruit for dessert.

- Low fat ricotta can also be used in cheesecakes or as a topping for fresh fruit.

7. Use high omega-3 and monounsaturated oils such as olive, peanut and canola oils

It is not necessary, or beneficial, to cut all fats out of your diet. In fact, some fat is essential for our health to provide essential fatty acids and for carrying fat soluble vitamins and anti-oxidants. This means that it is fine to use small amounts of oil in cooking and salad dressings but it is important to choose the right one. If you don't use oil you could also get these 'good' fats from eating nuts, seeds, avocado, olives and fish.

When choosing oil, you want to choose types which are high in monounsaturated and omega-3 fats. These include:

Olive oil is high in monounsaturated fats and low in saturates with a minimal polyunsaturated fat content, which is an advantage as it allows our bodies to make greater use of the omega-3 fats we obtain from other dietary sources, without any competition from excessive polyunsaturated omega-6 fats. Olive oil is also rich in antioxidants which have many health benefits. Olive oil can be used in cooking and is the best choice for salad dressings. Olive oil margarines are also available.

Peanut oil is a mild-tasting oil that oxidises slowly and can withstand high cooking temperatures. About 50 per cent of the fat in peanut oil is monounsaturated and another 30 per cent is polyunsaturated. This heart-healthy fat is good for Asian cooking such as stir-fries.

Canola oil, besides being high in monounsaturated fat, canola contains significant amounts of omega-3 fats. Canola oil is a multi-purpose cooking oil and can also be used for baking cakes and muffins. Margarine made from canola oil is also available.

Flaxseed oil (also known as linseed) is the richest plant source of omega-3s and contains very little omega-6 fats. But flaxseed oil is highly prone to oxidation (meaning the fats it contains turn rancid easily) so shouldn't be heated and needs to be stored carefully. It is best used in a salad dressing. Alternatively, linseeds can be freshly ground and sprinkled on cereal or added to cakes and muffins.

Cold pressed? Virgin? Extra virgin? Light? Extra light?

Cold pressed oils are those that have undergone minimal processing—this means that the oil is extracted from the seed, nut or fruit by mechanical pressing only, without heat or solvents. Cold pressed oils have a stronger flavour and colour than their regular counterparts, and they're also much richer in vitamin E (a natural preservative present in oils) and other antioxidants, giving them important health benefits. For example, extra-virgin olive oil—the best quality oil made from the first cold pressing of the olives—contains 30 to 40 different antioxidants. It is dark-coloured and strong in flavour.

Light and extra light oils are light in colour and flavour. The terms 'light' and 'extra light' don't mean, however, that the oil is lower in fat than any other oil—all oils are 100 per cent fat.

I was referred to the doctor for severe hypothyroidism. Although within a few weeks a thyroid hormone brought my thyroid tests to normal, I did not lose the weight I had put on and my periods remained really unpredictable. My GP ran serum prolactin, FSH and LH tests. The prolactin was abnormal, twice the upper limit of the normal range, but an MRI of the pituitary gland to diagnose (or exclude) a pituitary growth was inconclusive. Over the next few months the prolactin peaked again, and this time my doctor suspected that it may be linked to PCOS which an internal ultrasound scan confirmed. He prescribed metformin and at the same time I saw a dietitian who reviewed my diet and put me on a healthy low GI eating programme. I lost 6.2 kilograms (13½ pounds) in three weeks and have to say that I shouted from the rooftops that I have never eaten as much, nor felt as well ... All the energy that I thought I had lost has come back!
Juliet, 34

TYPES OF FAT AND THEIR SOURCES

There is less evidence to support reducing the amount of fat we eat than there is to recommend changing the type. Although foods contain a mixture of fatty acids, one type of fatty acid tends to predominate, allowing us to categorise foods according to their main fatty acid component. It is best to choose mono-unsaturated and polyunsaturated fats in place of saturated.

An asterisk next to a food in the following list means the food is a good source of omega-3 fatty acids.

Polyunsaturated products

Oils

Safflower, sunflower, grapeseed, soyabean*, corn, linseed*, cottonseed, walnut*, sesame, evening primrose oils

Spreads

Polyunsaturated margarines, tahini (sesame seed paste)

Nuts and seeds

Walnuts*, sunflower seeds, pumpkin seeds, sesame seeds

Other plant sources

Soyabeans, soya milk, wheat germ, wholegrains

Animal sources

Oily fish*

Monounsaturated products

Oils

Olive, canola (rapeseed), peanut, macadamia and mustard seed oils

Spreads

Olive oil margarines, peanut butter

Nuts and seeds

Cashews, macadamias, almonds, hazelnuts, pecans, pistachio, peanuts

Other plant sources
Avocado, olives

Animal sources
Very lean red meat, lean chicken, lean pork, egg yolks

Saturated products
Oils/Fats
Palm and palm kernel oil, coconut oil, drippings, lard, ghee, solid frying oils, cooking margarines and shortening

Spreads
Butter, cream cheese

Dairy foods
Full fat dairy products: cheese, cream, sour cream, yoghurt, full cream milk, ice-cream

Animal sources
Fat on beef, lamb, skin on chicken, sausage, salami, most luncheon meats

The flavour on fluids

An adequate fluid intake is essential for good health, but most people don't drink enough. Most adults need about 2 litres of fluid each day (about 8 glasses) to replace the fluid that is lost from the body. More is needed in hot weather, during exercise and if you work in air conditioning. An adequate fluid intake is important for kidney function, temperature regulation and for preventing constipation.

Water is the best fluid to quench your thirst and is also the best choice if you are watching your weight and insulin levels. Soft drinks, energy drinks and cordials contain large amounts of added sugar and it is best to avoid these where possible. Most fruit juices have a relatively low GI and can

SHOULD I AVOID ALL HIGH GI FOODS?

I am confused. Chocolate has a low GI and watermelon is high— does this mean I should choose chocolate over watermelon as a snack?

The GI of a food does not make it good or bad for us. High GI foods like potato and watermelon still make a valuable nutritional contribution to our diet. And low GI foods like pastry or chocolate that are high in saturated fat are no better for us because of their low GI. The nutritional benefits of different foods are many and varied, and it is advisable for you to base your food choices on the overall nutritional content of a food, particularly considering the saturated fat, salt, fibre and GI values.

be consumed in moderation but remember that they still contain a lot of carbohydrate from the natural fruit sugars. It would be better to eat the whole fruit (which still contains the fibre) rather than drinking the juice.

If you struggle to drink plain water you could try mineral or soda water with a slice of lemon or lime and a few fresh mint leaves. Or try diluting fruit juice with water, soda water or mineral water. Tea is also fine—green tea, in particular, has been shown to be high in antioxidants. If you like hot drinks, there are also a wide variety of herbal teas available but if you are pregnant you need to be careful as some types are not suitable during pregnancy.

Coffee and alcohol have a diuretic effect so should not be counted as part of your 8 glasses. Both are best consumed in moderation. Alcohol is also high in kilojoules so should be limited when watching your weight. The recommendations for women are for 1–2 alcoholic drinks per day with a few alcohol-free days per week.

Milk and soya milk are low GI but it is best to choose low fat varieties, particularly when weight loss is a goal. If you don't like the taste of milk or soya milk on their own, you could add a teaspoon of drinking chocolate for flavour, or make a fruit smoothie for a satisfying snack or breakfast on the run.

A quick guide to healthy low GI eating

If you are looking for ways to improve your diet, there are two important things to remember.

1. Identify the sources of carbohydrate in your diet and reduce high GI foods. Don't go to extremes; there is still room for your favourite high GI foods.

Some of the most common changes women tell us they have made to achieve a low GI diet are:

- swapping white and wholemeal breads for the grainy varieties

- choosing low GI breakfast cereals like oats

- eating more fruit and yoghurt in place of other snack foods

- adding more legumes to meals

- choosing more sweet potato, corn and pasta in place of white potato

2. Identify the sources of fat in your diet and look at ways you can reduce saturated fat. Choose monounsaturated and polyunsaturated fats, such as olive oil and sunflower oil, instead of saturated fats like butter and shortening. The body needs some fat, and there's room for your favourite fatty foods on occasion—just remember to watch your portions.

A few simple changes you could make to reduce your intake of saturated fat are:

- use avocado, hommous or nut spreads in place of butter

- choose lean meats and eat more fish and legumes in place of red meat

- choose low fat dairy products or try a calcium-fortified soya product instead

- snack on fruit, yoghurt, dried fruit and nuts, and hommous with vegetables in place of higher fat snack foods like chips, cakes and biscuits

Substituting high GI foods with low GI alternatives

High GI food	Low GI alternative
Bread—white or wholemeal	Bread containing lots of grains such as Burgen® or Vogels®—Soya and Linseed.
Processed breakfast cereals	Unrefined cereals such as rolled oats, oat bran or muesli or a low GI processed cereal like All Bran®.
Plain biscuits or crackers	Biscuits made with dried fruit, oats and wholegrains, oatcakes and Rich Tea biscuits.
Cakes and Muffins	Make them with fruit, oats and wholegrains
Potato	Substitute with baby new potatoes, sweet potato, sweetcorn, taro or yam
Rice	Try longer grain varieties such as basmati rice, or try pearled barley, noodles or wholegrain cereals instead

Putting it all together—a typical day the low GI way

We hope that having read this far you now have a good idea of how to build low GI foods into your diet. But just in case you're still not sure, it should look something like this:

Breakfast to get you going
Porridge with stewed apple, sultanas and low fat milk

Breakfast is the most important meal of the day—it gets your metabolism going and prevents you getting hungry and snacking on high fat foods later in the morning. Research has shown that people who eat breakfast regularly find it easier to lose weight and have better energy levels and concentration throughout the day. If you are always in a rush in the morning, it is well worth making the time for breakfast—5 or 10 minutes is all it takes.

Mid morning top-up
Apple or pear

There's nothing wrong with eating between meals if you are hungry. In fact, studies have shown that eating three meals and three snacks stimulates the body to use up more energy for metabolism than concentrating the same amount of food into three larger meals. Eating small regular meals and snacks will also help to keep your insulin levels lower.

Lunch to refuel
Tuna and three bean salad with pita bread

Taking a break for a satisfying lunchtime meal is important for maintaining energy levels and concentration and preventing hunger and excessive snacking during the afternoon and early evening. Whether you are eating at home, taking lunch with you or buying a meal out, there are plenty of healthy choices available.

Afternoon pick-me-up
Low fat yoghurt topped with a sprinkle of dried fruit and nuts

For many of the women we see, the afternoon is their 'danger time' when energy levels are low and hunger and sweet cravings begin. The key is to be organised and have a satisfying snack ready to prevent you heading for the work biscuit tin or buying a chocolate bar on the way home.

Dinner in minutes
Chicken and cashew nut stir-fry with hokkien noodles

When you are tired after a long day, it can be hard to get motivated to cook. Fortunately, putting a meal together at the end of the day doesn't have to take a lot of time and effort, as you will see with our recipes. The key is to have your kitchen well stocked with the right foods—use our shopping list to make sure you have everything you need.

A sweet treat
Berries with low fat ice-cream

If you feel like something sweet after dinner then go ahead. Fresh or canned fruits and low fat dairy products are the best choices as they are naturally sweet and most have a low GI.

Eating out

Many of the women we see comment that they find eating out difficult. We recognise that it can be harder when you don't have control over your food choices but there are many options which fit the low GI way of eating.

Try these:

- Asian: steamed, braised or stir-fried dishes with noodles

- Indian: Tandoori, dahl, vegetable and legume curries with basmati rice

- Mexican: tacos, burritos or tortillas with beans, salad, guacamole and a sprinkle of cheese (avoid the sour cream)

- Italian: small pasta with a tomato, pesto or seafood sauce served with a side salad

- pizza: gourmet style thin crust with vegetarian or seafood topping

- pita bread or felafel roll with hommous and tabbouli

- plain hamburger with lots of salad on a wholegrain roll (leave the butter)

- barbecue chicken (remove the skin) with a cob of corn and a side salad instead of chips

- Vietnamese rice paper rolls

While we suggest trying to include at least one low GI food with each meal, this may not always be possible when eating out. One option is to combine a high GI food with a low GI food to give a moderate effect—e.g. rice with legumes or potato with corn. If this is not possible, just have a small serve of the higher GI food and fill up with plenty of vegetables and salads. And, remember, if it is only once in a while it really won't matter. If you eat out a few times each week, you will need to be more careful.

Your healthy low GI shopping list

To make low GI choices easy choices, you need to stock your pantry with the right foods. Here are some ideas of what to include on your shopping list:

Breads
Burgen™ Soya and Linseed
Vogels® Soya and Linseed
Granary rye bread
Pumpernickel

Breakfast cereals
Rolled Oats (whole, not instant)
Oat Bran
All–Bran®
Natural muesli

Rice, pasta and grains
Basmati rice
Pasta—fresh or dried
Noodles
Pearl barley
Cracked wheat
Quinoa

Legumes
Dried legumes e.g. lentils, split peas, chickpeas, kidney beans, cannellini beans
Canned legumes, e.g. kidney beans, three or four bean mix
Baked beans
Mexican style beans

Vegetables
All fresh, frozen and canned vegetables
All salad vegetables
Canned tomatoes
Sweet potato, corn, yam, baby new potato, taro

Fruits
All fruits are suitable but the lowest GI varieties include:

Apples	Grapefruit	Grapes	Kiwi fruit
Oranges	Pears	Plums	Peaches

Dried fruit including apricots, sultanas, apples, prunes and pears
Canned fruits in natural juice
Fruit snack packs
Fruit juices (limited to 1–2 glasses per day)

Meats
Lean cuts such as trim beef, lamb, veal and pork
Skinless chicken or turkey
Low fat mince
Lean deli meats such as ham, corned beef, pastrami, turkey and chicken breast

Fish and seafood
All fresh fish
Canned fish including salmon, sardines, tuna, mackerel and herring
Smoked fish such as smoked cod and smoked salmon
Frozen fish products without crumbs or made with poly- or monounsaturated oils (check the label)
Most seafood except battered or crumbed

Dairy foods or non-dairy alternatives
Reduced fat or skimmed milk
Calcium-fortified soya milk

Low fat or no fat yoghurts
Soya yoghurts
UHT or powdered skimmed milk for cooking
Canned evaporated skimmed milk
Low fat ice-cream or soya ice-cream
Cottage cheese, low fat ricotta cheese
Low fat flavoured milks or soya milks
Low fat cheese: block, slices or grated for cooking

Spreads
If you use a spread, choose one labelled 'polyunsaturated' or 'monounsaturated', and preferably one that is salt reduced. Alternatively try using avocado, hommous, tahini (sesame seed spread) or nut butters—these contain good types of fats as well as providing a variety of vitamins and minerals.

Flavours, sauces, oils and dressings
Fresh and dried herbs
Spices
Cold pressed olive oil, canola or peanut oil
Vinegar: white wine, red wine and balsamic
Curry powders and pastes
Bottled tomato pasta sauces and tomato paste
Sauces including soya, oyster, sweet chilli, hoisin and fish
Bottled minced ginger, garlic and chilli
Black pepper
Mustard
Sundried tomatoes, olives, artichoke hearts

Your low GI menus

Armed with the information in this book we hope you will be able to make the switch to the healthy low GI way of eating with ease. But, as we know from the women we see, some of you like more direction. You want to know exactly what you should be eating from day to day and from meal to meal. Keeping this in mind, we have designed some sample healthy summer and winter menus which you could use to give you ideas or which you may wish to follow for a few weeks to get started on a low GI way of eating.

The menus follow our 7 dietary guidelines and emphasise fruits, vegetables, legumes, wholegrain and low GI breads and cereals, lean meats and seafood, low fat dairy products and healthy oils. They also incorporate the recipes we have included in this book, which are marked with an asterisk (*).

We have not included serving sizes as everyone has different energy needs and appetites. Start by focusing on making healthier food choices rather than worrying about amounts, and if you need more specific advice we suggest that you see a Registered Dietitian (details of how to contact an RD can be found on page 47).

Low GI Summer Menu

	Breakfast	Morning snack	Lunch
MONDAY	Low fat toasted muesli*	Fruit	Garden salad with sliced chicken breast
TUESDAY	All-Bran™ with strawberries and low fat milk	2 sweet oat biscuits	Wholemeal pita bread with hommous, salad and felafel
WEDNESDAY	Granary toast with avocado and tomato	Fruit	Greek salad with low fat feta and olives
THURSDAY	Low fat toasted muesli* with yoghurt	Handful of roasted chickpeas	Granary sandwich with chicken, avocado and salad
FRIDAY	Cooked oat porridge with sliced banana and low fat milk	Fruit	Salad with tuna and four bean mix with a granary roll
SATURDAY	Sourdough French toast with peaches*	Fruit	Chickpea and Beetroot Salad*
SUNDAY	Granary toast with poached egg and grilled tomato	Fruit	Granary roll with chickpea burger, salad and sweet chilli sauce

Afternoon snack	Dinner	Dessert
Handful of raw nuts	Tomato and salmon pasta* with salad	Fresh fruit
Low fat yoghurt	Balsamic lamb* with sweet potato mash, steamed beans and baby squash	Poached pears in cranberry *
2 wholegrain crispbreads with ricotta and tomato	Bean and Corn Burritos*	Fresh fruit salad
Berries and low fat yoghurt	Fish and white bean salsa and salad*	Cherry strudel*
Granary roll with ricotta and tomato	Chargrilled beef with Thai noodle salad	Hot chocolate with low fat milk or soya milk
Hommous with baked wholemeal pita bread, carrot and celery	Tandoori chicken* with basmati rice	Handful of dried fruit and nuts
Low fat fruit smoothie	Creamy mustard pork* with red cabbage	Baked ricotta cheesecake*

Low GI Winter Menu

	Breakfast	Morning Tea	Lunch
MONDAY	Mixed grain porridge with dried fruit compote and yoghurt*	Fruit	Granary toasted sandwich with ricotta and tomato
TUESDAY	Granary toast with baked beans	Fruit	Wholemeal pita bread with hommous, chicken and tabbouli
WEDNESDAY	Low fat toasted muesli with low fat milk or yoghurt	Fruit	Thick vegetable soup*
THURSDAY	Fruit loaf with ricotta	Handful of dried fruit and nuts	Granary chicken, avocado and tomato toasted sandwich
FRIDAY	Porridge with stewed apple and low fat milk	Fruit	Tuna and bean salad with garlic pita toasts*
SATURDAY	Ricotta blueberry hotcakes*	Fruit	Minestrone soup
SUNDAY	Sweetcorn, bacon and mushroom omelettes* with soya and linseed toast	Fruit	Lamb burgers with sweet potato wedges, salsa and salad*

Afternoon Tea	Dinner	Dessert
Fruit Loaf with ricotta	Mediterranean chicken* with spiral pasta* and broccoli	Honey oat biscuits*
Ryvita™ crispbreads with avocado and tomato	Lentil and ricotta cannelloni* with green salad	Fruit salad with yoghurt
Pear and chocolate muffins*	Lamb cutlets with pea pilaf*	Low fat hot chocolate
Berries and low fat yoghurt	Pasta with feta and roasted vegetables*	Apple and rhubarb crumble*
Choc nut biscotti*	Tofu and vegetable noodles*	Tinned fruit and custard
Salsa with baked pita bread, carrot, and celery	Slow cooked pork and vegetables* with steamed greens	Fragrant rice pudding with plums*
Low fat yoghurt	Wholemeal pita bread pizzas	Fresh fruit

CHAPTER 5

RECIPES

Breakfasts
Quick and easy light meals
Main meals
Desserts and sweet treats

BREAKFASTS

Mixed Grain Porridge with Dried Fruit Compote and Yoghurt

Per serve:	
1097 kJ/258 Cal	Protein 9 g
Fat 2.5 g	Carbohydrate 50 g
Saturated fat 0.5 g	GI Low

Preparation time: 10 minutes
Cooking time: 15 minutes

- 50 g (2 oz) dried apples
- 50 g (2 oz) dried apricots
- 50 g (2 oz) pitted prunes
- 1 litre (1¾ pints) water
- 1 cinnamon stick
- 75 g (3 oz) rolled oats
- 100 g (3 oz) rolled barley
- 200 g (6 oz) low fat vanilla yoghurt, to serve

1. Combine the apples, apricots, prunes, 250 ml (8½ fl oz) of water and the cinnamon stick in a medium–sized saucepan. Bring to the boil, then reduce the heat, partially cover and simmer for 10–15 minutes, or until the fruit is soft. Discard the cinnamon stick and cool slightly.
2. Meanwhile, place the oats and barley in another medium-sized saucepan and add 750 ml (25½ fl oz) of water. Bring to the boil, then reduce the heat and simmer for 3–5 minutes, stirring frequently, until creamy.
3. Spoon the porridge into serving bowls, top with the fruit compote and drizzle with some of the fruit cooking liquid. Add a dollop of yoghurt and serve immediately.

Serves 4

Note: The compote can be made up to three days in advance. Refrigerate until required, then reheat, or serve cold.

Natural Toasted Muesli

While this muesli is relatively high in fat, most of it comes
from the 'healthy' fats in the nuts and seeds.

Per serve:	
1292 kJ/304 Cal	Protein 9 g
Fat 12 g	Carbohydrate 41 g
Saturated fat 1 g	GI Low

Preparation time: 15 minutes
Cooking time: 30 minutes (plus 30 minutes' cooling time)

250 g (10 oz) rolled oats
270 g (11 oz) rolled rye
60 g (2½ oz) raw unsalted pumpkin seeds
50 g (2 oz) sunflower seeds
35 g (1 oz) almonds, chopped
35 g (1 oz) hazelnuts, chopped
185 g (7 oz) dried apricots, chopped
125 g (5 oz) sultanas

1. Preheat the oven to 180°C (350°F/gas mark 4).
2. Place the oats, rye, pumpkin and sunflower seeds and
   nuts in a large baking dish and mix until well
   combined.
3. Bake for 35 minutes, until lightly toasted, stirring
   several times during cooking.
4. Cool completely, then stir in the apricots and sultanas.
   Serve with low fat milk or yoghurt, and fresh fruit in
   season. Keep the muesli in an airtight container and
   store in a cool, dark place for up to one month.

Serves 12

Sourdough French Toast with Peaches

Per serve:

960 kJ/226 Cal	Protein 12 g
Fat 5.5 g	Carbohydrate 31 g
Saturated fat 1.5 g	GI Low

Preparation time: 10 minutes
Cooking time: 8 minutes

2 eggs
250 ml (10 fl oz) low fat milk
1 tablespoon maple syrup
pinch nutmeg
olive oil spray
4 slices of wholemeal sourdough, each about 2 cm
    thick
4 fresh peaches, sliced

1. Whisk the eggs, milk, maple syrup and nutmeg
   together in a shallow bowl. Lightly spray a non-stick
   frypan and heat over a medium heat.
2. Dip the bread in the egg mixture and turn to coat
   completely. Place the bread in the heated pan and
   cook for 2–3 minutes on each side until golden
   brown. Set aside and keep warm.
3. Spray the pan lightly again, and cook the peach slices
   for 1–2 minutes on each side, until just softened. Serve
   the French toast topped with the peaches.

Serves 4

Ricotta Blueberry Hotcakes

Keep cooked hotcakes warm on a plate covered with foil in a very low oven (about 120°C (250°F, gas mark 1)) while cooking the remaining batter.

Per serve:	
1113 kJ/262 Cal	Protein 15 g
Fat 8 g	Carbohydrate 32 g
Saturated fat 3.5 g	GI Moderate/Medium

Preparation time: 10 minutes
Cooking time: 7 minutes

> 150 g (6 oz) reduced fat fresh ricotta
> 2 eggs, separated
> 125 ml (5 fl oz) low fat milk
> 2 tablespoons caster sugar
> 1 teaspoon vanilla essence
> 80 g (3 oz) stoneground wholemeal flour
> 2 teaspoons baking powder
> 155 g (6 oz) fresh or frozen blueberries
> olive oil spray
> 200 g (8 oz) low fat vanilla yoghurt, to serve

1. Place the ricotta in a large mixing bowl and mash with a fork. Add the egg yolks, milk, sugar and vanilla and mix with a wooden spoon to combine. Add the flour and baking powder and fold in with a large metal spoon or rubber spatula until just combined. Do not overbeat.
2. Beat the egg whites with an electric beater until firm peaks form, then gently fold into the ricotta mixture, along with the blueberries.
3. Spray a large non-stick frypan lightly with oil, and heat over a low heat. Drop ¼ cupfuls of the batter into the pan, and cook for 2 minutes, until golden underneath. Turn and cook a further 1½ minutes, until

the hotcakes have risen and are golden brown and cooked through. Repeat with the remaining batter, to make 8 hotcakes. Serve immediately with dollops of yoghurt.

Serves 4

Sweetcorn and Mushroom Omelette

Per serve:

1216 kJ/286 Cal	Protein 22 g
Fat 17 g	Carbohydrate 25 g
Saturated fat 4 g	GI Low

Preparation time: 10 minutes
Cooking time: 10 minutes

> olive oil spray
> 100 g (4 oz) button mushrooms, sliced
> 1 × 300 g (12 oz) can corn kernels, well drained
> 15 g (½ oz) flatleaf parsley, finely chopped
> 6 eggs
> 4 slices Burgen® Soya and Linseed Bread, toasted
> ½ small avocado

1. Lightly spray a 30 cm non-stick frypan with olive oil. Cook the mushrooms on low heat for 2 minutes, or until soft.
2. Combine the mushrooms, corn and parsley in a bowl. In a jug or bowl whisk 3 of the eggs until lightly beaten. Pour into the frypan, and cook over a medium heat for 2 minutes, until almost set.
3. Sprinkle half the corn mixture over half of the omelette surface, and fold over to enclose. Cook for a further 2–3 minutes, then cut the omelette in half using a non-scratch spatula. Repeat with remaining ingredients. Spread the toast with avocado, and serve with the omelette.

Serves 4

QUICK AND EASY LIGHT MEALS
(on the table in around 30 minutes)

Tuna and Bean Salad with Garlic Pita Toasts

Per serve:

1445 kJ/340 Cal	Protein 25 g
Fat 8 g	Carbohydrate 36 g
Saturated fat 1 g	GI Low

Preparation time: 10 minutes
Cooking time: 2–3 minutes

> 1 × 185 g (7 oz) can tuna, drained and flaked
> 1 small red onion, very finely sliced
> 2 ripe tomatoes, cut into thin wedges
> 1 × 400 g (16 oz) can cannellini beans, rinsed and
>   drained
> 1 bunch rocket, trimmed and leaves torn
> 2 tablespoons lemon juice
> 1 tablespoon extra-virgin olive oil
> salt and freshly ground black pepper, to taste
> 4 small wholemeal pita breads
> 1 large garlic clove, peeled and halved

1. Combine the tuna, onion, tomatoes, beans and rocket
   in a large bowl. Drizzle with lemon juice and olive oil,
   season with salt and pepper and toss gently to combine.
2. Toast the pita bread on both sides, then rub the cut
   garlic clove all over one side. Break into pieces, and
   serve with the salad.

Serves 4

Bean and Corn Burritos

This makes a delicious lunch to take to work. Store the bean mixture in an airtight container, and the lettuce and cheese in another. One option is to use wholemeal lavash bread in place of the tortillas, then assemble just before eating.

Per serve:

1835 kJ/434 Cal	Protein 21 g
Fat 12 g	Carbohydrate 60 g
Saturated fat 4.5 g	GI Low

Preparation time: 10 minutes
Cooking time: 5 minutes

1 × 400 g (16 oz) can corn kernels, drained
1 × 400 g (16 oz) can red kidney beans, rinsed and
    drained
2 large ripe tomatoes, chopped
2 shallots, finely sliced
75 g (3 oz) taco sauce
4 × 16 cm white corn tortillas
4 large iceberg lettuce leaves, shredded
90 g (4 oz) reduced fat cheese, grated

1. Preheat the oven to 180°C (350°F/gas mark 4).
2. Combine the corn, beans, tomatoes, shallots and taco sauce in a bowl.
3. Wrap the tortillas in foil and warm in the oven for 5 minutes.
4. To assemble, spread a lettuce leaf over a warmed tortilla, and top with the bean mixture and grated cheese. Fold the bottom of the tortilla over the filling, and roll up to enclose. Serve immediately.

Serves 4

Chargrilled Beef with Thai Noodle Salad

Per serve:

1135 kJ/267 Cal	Protein 31 g
Fat 11.5 g	Carbohydrate 9 g
Saturated fat 3.5 g	GI Low

Preparation time: 25 minutes
Cooking time: 10 minutes

50 g (2 oz) dried rice vermicelli
1 carrot, peeled and cut into thin strips
1 cucumber, cut into thin strips
1 red pepper, cut into thin strips
1 large handful of bean sprouts
1 bunch mint, leaves picked and torn
1 bunch coriander, leaves only
1½ tablespoons (30 ml) lime juice
1 tablespoon (20 ml) fish sauce
1 tablespoon (20 ml) peanut oil
1 teaspoon caster sugar
1 small fresh red chilli, finely chopped
4 fillet beef steaks (about 125 g (5 oz) each)
1 teaspoon peanut oil, extra
freshly ground black pepper, to taste

1. Place the rice vermicelli in a bowl and cover with plenty of cold water. Set aside for 5 minutes, or until the noodles become translucent. Drain well and cut into short lengths.
2. Place the vermicelli, carrot, cucumber, red pepper, bean sprouts, mint and coriander in a large serving bowl. Toss well to combine.
3. Whisk the lime juice, fish sauce, peanut oil, sugar and chilli together.
4. Preheat a chargrill on medium–high. If you don't have a chargrill you can use a heavy-based frypan.

Brush the steaks with the extra peanut oil and season with black pepper. Cook for 3 minutes on each side, or to your liking. Set aside for 5 minutes.

5. Add the dressing to the salad and toss to coat. Serve the noodle salad with the steaks.

Serves 4

Chargrilled Fish with White Bean Salsa

This white bean salsa can be made ahead of time and kept in the refrigerator until you are ready to serve. For a change, try it with chargrilled chicken, or as a light meal on its own with rye bread.

Per serve:	
1160 kJ/273 Cal	Protein 33 g
Fat 17.5 g	Carbohydrate 11 g
Saturated fat 2.5 g	GI Low

Preparation time: 15 minutes
Cooking time: 10 minutes

4 × 100 g (4 oz) firm white-fleshed fish cutlets, such as cod
1 teaspoon (5 ml) olive oil

White bean salsa

1 × 400 g (16 oz) can white beans, rinsed and drained
2 ripe tomatoes, finely chopped
3 shallots, thinly sliced
25 g (1 oz) fresh coriander leaves, shredded
1½ tablespoons (30 ml) fresh lime juice
1 tablespoon (20 ml) extra-virgin olive oil
salt and freshly ground black pepper, to taste

To serve

80 g (3½ oz) mixed salad leaves (mesclun)
2 tablespoons vinaigrette dressing (see recipe below)

1. To make the salsa, place the beans, tomatoes, shallots, coriander, lime juice and olive oil in a small bowl and toss lightly to combine. Season well with salt and pepper and set aside while you prepare the fish.
2. Preheat a chargrill on medium–high. If you don't have a chargrill, use a heavy-based frypan.
3. Brush both sides of the fish with olive oil and season

with salt and pepper. Chargrill the fish for 3–4
minutes on each side, or until cooked. The fish is ready
when it flakes gently when tested with a fork. Serve
with the salsa, salad and a light vinaigrette dressing.

Serves 4

Cook's tip
Mesclun is simply a mix of fresh, tender young salad
leaves and may include a variety of lettuces such as
iceberg, cos, mignonette and oakleaf, plus baby spinach
leaves, rocket, curly endive, broadleaf endive, nasturtium,
snowpea shoots, raddicchio and sometimes edible flowers.
You can buy it ready-made in most supermarkets, or mix
your own to taste.

Vinaigrette dressing
In a screw-top jar combine 2 tablespoons olive oil with
the juice of 1 lemon, 1 tablespoon of white wine vinegar,
a clove of crushed garlic and one teaspoon of grainy
mustard. Add 1 tablespoon of finely chopped continental
parsley, 1 small tomato that has been very finely diced and
3 to 4 finely diced pitted black olives. Shake to combine.
Stand about 30 minutes before serving. Serves 8.

Chickpea and Beetroot Salad

Per serve:	
1679 kJ/395 Cal	Protein 20 g
Fat 11.5 g	Carbohydrate 54 g
Saturated fat 1.5 g	GI Low

Preparation time: 20 minutes

> 2 × 400 g (16 oz) cans chickpeas, rinsed and drained
> 1 red onion, cut into thin wedges
> 100 g (4 oz) baby rocket leaves
> 1 tablespoon (20 ml) extra-virgin olive oil
> 1½ tablespoons (30 ml) red wine vinegar
> 1½ tablespoons (30 ml) lemon juice
> 1 clove garlic, crushed
> pinch caster sugar
> salt and freshly ground black pepper, to taste
> 1 × 450 g (18 oz) can beetroot wedges, drained and
>   patted dry with paper towel
> 4 slices granary bread

1. Place the chickpeas, onion and rocket in a large serving bowl.
2. Whisk the olive oil, vinegar, lemon juice, garlic and sugar. Season with salt and pepper.
3. Add the dressing to the salad and toss gently to combine. Then add the beetroot and toss gently again. Serve with the bread.

Serves 4

Tomato Fettuccine with Salmon and Baby Spinach

Per serve:	
2023 kJ/476 Cal	Protein 33 g
Fat 15.5 g	Carbohydrate 45 g
Saturated fat 6.5 g	GI Low

Preparation time: 10 minutes
Cooking time: 10 minutes

> 3 teaspoons (15 ml) extra-virgin olive oil
> 1 large red onion, cut into thin wedges
> 65 g (2½ oz) capers, drained and patted dry with paper towel
> 2 cloves garlic, crushed
> 4 large ripe tomatoes, chopped
> 80 ml (3 oz) vegetable stock
> 500 g (20 oz) fresh fettuccine
> 80 g (3 oz) baby spinach leaves
> 1 × 415 g (16¼ oz) can red salmon, bones and skin removed, broken into large pieces
> 2 tablespoons (40 ml) fresh lemon juice
> salt and freshly ground black pepper, to taste

1. Heat the oil in a large frypan over a medium heat. Add the onion, capers and garlic and cook, stirring often, for 6–7 minutes or until the onion softens. Add the tomatoes and stir for 1 minute. Add the stock and increase the heat to high. Bring to the boil then remove from the heat.
2. Meanwhile, cook the pasta in a large saucepan of salted water for 2–3 minutes or until tender. Drain well and return to the pan.
3. Add the onion mixture and spinach leaves to the pasta. Toss well until combined and the spinach starts

to wilt. Add the salmon and lemon juice. Toss gently and season to taste. Serve immediately.

Serves 4

Cook's tip

Most types of pasta have a similar GI, so spaghetti or spirali, for example, could also be used in this recipe.

Pork with Creamy Mustard Sauce

Per serve:

1322 kJ/311 Cal	Protein 41 g
Fat 9 g	Carbohydrate 17 g
Saturated fat 2 g	GI Low

Preparation time: 10 minutes
Cooking time: 20 minutes

> 1 tablespoon (20 ml) olive oil
> 600 g (about ¼) red cabbage, thinly sliced
> 2 carrots, grated
> 1 onion, cut into thin wedges
> 125 ml (5 fl oz) chicken stock
> 4 pork cutlets (about 150 g each (5½ oz)), trimmed of excess fat
> 250 ml (10 fl oz) orange juice
> 125 ml (5 fl oz) light evaporated milk
> 1 tablespoon wholegrain mustard
> 25 g (1 oz) chopped fresh dill
> salt and freshly ground black pepper, to taste

1. Heat half the oil in a large, heavy-based saucepan over a medium heat. Add the cabbage, carrots and onion. Cook, stirring, for 3 minutes. Add the stock, cover and reduce the heat to low. Cook for 15 minutes, or until the vegetables are tender.
2. Meanwhile, heat the remaining oil in a large, heavy-based frypan over a medium heat. Add the pork cutlets and cook for 4 minutes on each side. Transfer to a plate, cover loosely with foil and set aside.
3. Increase the pan heat to high and add the orange juice, evaporated milk and mustard. Bring to the boil, stirring. Boil uncovered for 6–7 minutes, stirring often, until the sauce reduces and thickens slightly. Return the cutlets to the pan and turn to coat in the sauce.

4. Stir the dill into the cabbage mixture and season well.
    To serve, spoon the sauce over the cutlets and
    accompany with the vegetables.

Serves 4

Tofu and Vegetable Noodles

Per serve:

1620 kJ/381 Cal	Protein 19 g
Fat 14 g	Carbohydrate 44 g
Saturated fat 1.5 g	GI Low

Preparation time: 10 minutes (plus 4 hours for marinating)
Cooking time: 15 minutes

80 ml (3 fl oz) soya sauce
60 ml (2 fl oz) oyster sauce
60 ml (2 fl oz) hoisin sauce
2 cloves garlic, crushed
1 × 375 g (15 oz) packet firm tofu, drained and cut
    into 3 cm pieces
1 × 450 g packet hokkein noodles
1½ tablespoons (30 ml) olive oil
1 onion, cut into thin wedges
1 red pepper, cut into thin strips
200 g (8 oz) baby aubergine, thinly sliced lengthways
1 × 225 g (11 oz) can bamboo shoot slices, drained
2 tablespoons (40 ml) water

1. Combine the soya, oyster and hoisin sauce with the
   garlic in a shallow glass dish. Add the tofu and turn
   to coat in the marinade. Cover and refrigerate for
   4 hours, turning once.
2. Place the noodles in a large heatproof bowl and
   cover with boiling water. Set aside for 5 minutes then
   drain well.
3. Heat 2 teaspoons of the oil in a wok over a high heat.
   Add the onion, pepper and aubergine. Stir-fry for
   2–3 minutes, or until the vegetables are almost tender.
   Toss in the bamboo shoots. Add the water, cover and
   cook for 1–2 minutes. Transfer the vegetables to a
   bowl.

4. Wipe out the wok. Add the remaining oil and heat over a high heat. Drain the tofu, reserving the marinade. Stir-fry the tofu for 2–3 minutes, or until golden. Return the vegetables to the wok and add the reserved marinade and noodles. Toss for 1–2 minutes, or until well combined and heated through. Serve immediately.

Serves 4

MAIN MEALS
to take a bit of time over . . .

Thick Vegetable Soup

The dried soup mix in this recipe is a combination of barley, red lentils and split peas. Some brands also contain dried beans, in which case add another 15–20 minutes to the cooking time. This type of mix is available from supermarkets or health food shops. The cooled soup may be packed into airtight containers and frozen for up to three months. Freeze in single serves to make handy lunches.

Per serve:	
510 kJ/120 Cal	Protein 7 g
Fat 2 g	Carbohydrate 18 g
Saturated fat 0.5 g	GI Low

Preparation time: 20 minutes
Cooking time: 1 hour

> 2 teaspoons olive oil
> 1 onion, chopped
> 2 carrots, chopped
> 2 celery sticks, sliced
> 200 g (8 oz) dried soup mix
> 2 litres (3½ pints) vegetable stock
> 1 × 400 g can (16 oz) chopped tomatoes
> 2 courgettes, chopped
> 3 tablespoons chopped flat leaf parsley

1. Heat the oil in a large saucepan, and add the onion, carrot and celery. Cook over a medium heat for 5 minutes, stirring occasionally, until the onion has softened.
2. Add the soup mix, stock and tomatoes. Cover and bring to the boil, then reduce the heat to medium–low. Tilt the lid slightly, and cook for 30 minutes.

3. Add the courgettes and cook for a further 30 minutes, until all the ingredients are tender. Serve sprinkled with parsley.

Serves 8

Lamb Cutlets with Pea Pilaf

Per serve:

1785 kJ/420 Cal	Protein 43 g
Fat 12.5 g	Carbohydrate 34 g
Saturated fat 4.5 g	GI Mod

Preparation time: 15 minutes (plus 1 hour for marinating)
Cooking time: 30 minutes

125 g (5 oz) plain low fat yoghurt
1 teaspoon ground coriander
1 teaspoon ground cumin
2 teaspoons freshly grated ginger
8 lean lamb cutlets

Pea pilaf
2 teaspoons canola oil
1 small onion, halved and sliced
4 cardamom pods, lightly crushed
½ teaspoon ground turmeric
135 g (5½ oz) basmati rice
200 g cauliflower (½ small head), cut into small florets
250 ml (10 fl oz) vegetable stock
1 head broccoli (about 350 g (12½ oz)), cut into small florets
150 g (6 oz) fresh or frozen green peas

1. Combine the yoghurt with the coriander, cumin and ginger. Place the lamb cutlets in a non-metallic dish and spread the yoghurt mixture over the meat section of the cutlets. Cover and refrigerate for 1 hour.
2. To make the pilaf, heat the oil in a large saucepan, and add the onion. Cook over a medium heat for 3–5 minutes, stirring often, until the onion is soft and lightly golden. Add the cardamom pods, turmeric and rice, and cook, stirring, for 30 seconds.
3. Add the cauliflower and stock, stir once, then cover

and bring to the boil. Reduce the heat to very low, and cook tightly covered for 10 minutes. Add the broccoli and peas and cook for a further 10 minutes. Remove from the heat and stand, still covered, for five minutes.

4. Meanwhile, heat a chargrill or non-stick frypan, and cook the lamb over a medium–high heat for 3 minutes on each side, or to your liking. Serve the lamb cutlets with the rice pilaf.

Serves 4

Pasta with Roasted Vegetables and Feta

Per serve:	
1670 kJ/393 Cal	Protein 18 g
Fat 6 g	Carbohydrate 65 g
Saturated fat 2.5 g	GI Low

Preparation time: 20 minutes
Cooking time: 45 minutes

1 small red onion, peeled and cut into wedges
1 red pepper, cut into 3 cm pieces
2 Roma tomatoes, quartered lengthways
200 g (8 oz) sweet potato, peeled and cut into 2 cm
    chunks
1 small aubergine, cut into 2 cm chunks
olive oil spray
300 g (12 oz) short pasta, such as penne or spirals
100 g (4 oz) reduced fat feta, crumbled
15 g (½ oz) basil leaves, shredded
1 small garlic clove, crushed (optional)

1. Preheat the oven to 180°C (350°F/gas mark 4).
2. Spread the onion, pepper, tomatoes, sweet potato and
   aubergine on two large oven trays, spray lightly with
   oil and toss the vegetables to coat. Roast for about 45
   minutes, until tender and browned.
3. When the vegetables are almost ready, cook the pasta
   in a large saucepan of boiling water, according to the
   packet directions, until *al dente*. Drain well and return
   to the pan. Add the vegetables, feta, basil and garlic and
   toss to combine. Serve immediately.

Serves 4

Lentil and Ricotta Cannelloni

Per serve:

1439 kJ/339 Cal	Protein 25 g
Fat 11.5 g	Carbohydrate 33 g
Saturated fat 5.7 g	GI Low

Preparation time: 30 minutes
Cooking time: 1 hour

> 2 teaspoons olive oil
> 1 small onion, finely chopped
> 2 garlic cloves, crushed
> 1 × 400 g (12 oz) can chopped tomatoes
> 250 ml (9 fl oz) vegetable stock
> 250 g (10 oz) red lentils
> 1 bunch (450 g (15½ oz)) English spinach, stems
>   trimmed
> salt and freshly ground black pepper, to taste
> 4 fresh lasagne sheets (16 × 30 cm)
> 400 g (12 oz) reduced fat fresh ricotta
> pinch nutmeg
> 500 ml (18 fl oz) Italian tomato cooking sauce
> 60 g (2½ oz) grated reduced fat cheddar cheese

1. Preheat the oven to 200°C (400°F/gas mark 6).
2. Heat the oil in a large saucepan, and cook the onion over a low heat for 5 minutes, until soft. Add the garlic and stir for a further 30 seconds, then add the tomatoes, stock and lentils. Bring to the boil, reduce the heat to low and simmer for 20 minutes, covered, until the lentils are tender. Stir occasionally to prevent the mixture from catching on the bottom of the pan.
3. Roughly chop the spinach leaves and stir into the lentil mixture to wilt. Season the mixture with salt and pepper, then cool to room temperature.
4. Meanwhile, cut each lasagne sheet crossways into three pieces. Mash the ricotta in a bowl with the nutmeg

until smooth. Then spread 250 ml (9 fl oz) of the tomato sauce over the base of a large lasagne dish.

5. Spread a generous tablespoon of the lentil mixture along the centre of a lasagne piece. Spoon 1 heaped tablespoon of ricotta over the lentil mixture. Roll up to enclose, and place seam side down in the lasagne dish. Repeat with the remaining ingredients, fitting them snugly into the dish. Pour the remaining tomato sauce over to cover, and sprinkle with cheese. Bake for 35 minutes, until the pasta is tender. Serve with a green salad.

Serves 6

Tandoori Chicken with Herbed Rice

Per serve:	
1786 kJ/420 Cal	Protein 42 g
Fat 4.5 g	Carbohydrate 51 g
Saturated fat 1 g	GI Moderate/Medium

Preparation time: 15 minutes (plus 6–8 hours for
marinating)
Cooking time: 20 minutes

130 g (5 oz) tandoori paste★
2 tablespoons low fat natural yoghurt, plus 130 g
(5 oz) for serving
2 tablespoons (40 ml) lemon juice
4 (about 125 g/5 oz each) single skinless chicken
breast fillets
200 g (8 oz) basmati rice
25 g (1 oz) fresh coriander leaves, finely shredded
25 g (1 oz) fresh mint leaves, finely shredded
rind of 1 small lime, finely grated
¼ small cucumber, finely chopped
2 ripe tomatoes, finely chopped
½ small red onion, finely chopped
pappadums, cooked following microwave packet
instructions
100 g (4 oz) mango chutney

1. Combine the tandoori paste, yoghurt and 1 tablespoon
lemon juice in a shallow glass or ceramic dish. Use a
sharp knife to make 3 slits (about 1 cm deep) in each
chicken breast. Add the chicken to the tandoori
mixture. Spoon the paste all over the chicken, pushing
it into the slits. Cover and place in the refrigerator for
6–8 hours to marinate.
2. Preheat the oven to 200°C (400°F/gas mark 6). Place
the marinated chicken on a wire rack over a large

baking dish and bake for 20 minutes, or until the chicken is cooked.

3. Meanwhile, cook the rice in a large saucepan of boiling water for 10–12 minutes or until tender. Drain well and return to the pan. Set aside for 5 minutes. Add the coriander, mint and lime rind to the rice and toss to combine.

4. Combine the extra yoghurt and cucumber in a small serving bowl and mix together the tomato, onion and remaining lemon juice in a separate bowl.

5. Serve the chicken with the herbed rice, cucumber yoghurt, tomato salsa, pappadums and chutney.

Serves 4

★ Available in supermarkets

Lamb Burgers with Sweet Potato Chips and Spinach Salad

Per serve:	
1984 kJ/467 Cal	Protein 27 g
Fat 11 g	Carbohydrate 39 g
Saturated fat 2.5 g	GI Low

Preparation time: 20 minutes
Cooking time: 50 minutes

Sweet potato chips
1¼ kg sweet potato, peeled and cut into thick chips
1 tablespoon olive oil
salt and freshly ground black pepper, to taste

Lamb burgers
500 g (17½ oz) extra lean lamb mince
60 g (2½ oz) fresh breadcrumbs, made from Bürgen®
    Soya and Linseed Bread
25 g (1 oz) fresh parsley, finely chopped
25 g (1 oz) fresh mint, finely chopped
1 egg
1 clove garlic, crushed
½ tablespoon olive oil

Spinach salad
100 g (4 oz) baby spinach leaves
200 g (8 oz) punnet cherry tomatoes
1 tablespoon fresh lemon juice
freshly ground black pepper, to taste

To serve
1 × 320 g (13 oz) jar mild tomato salsa dip

1. Preheat the oven to 220°C (425°F/gas mark 7) and
    line two large baking trays with non-stick baking
    paper.
2. To make the chips, place the sweet potato, olive oil,

salt and pepper in a large bowl and toss well to coat. Spread the sweet potato over the lined trays in a single layer. Bake for 45–50 minutes, swapping trays around once, until cooked through and crisp.

3. Meanwhile, to make the burgers, place the mince, breadcrumbs, parsley, mint, egg and garlic in a large bowl. Use clean hands to mix until well combined. Divide the mixture into six portions and shape each into a round patty. Heat the olive oil in a large frypan over a medium heat. Add the patties and cook for 4–5 minutes on each side, or until cooked through.

4. To make the spinach salad, combine the spinach, tomatoes, lemon juice and pepper in a small serving bowl.

5. Serve the burgers with the sweet potato chips, salad and salsa.

Serves 6

Slow-cooked Pork and Vegetables

Per serve:

1530 kJ/360 Cal	Protein 39 g
Fat 11.5 g	Carbohydrate 18 g
Saturated fat 2.5 g	GI Moderate/Medium

Preparation time: 15 minutes
Cooking time: 1 hour, 45 minutes

> 1 kg (2.2 lbs) pork neck, cut into 4 cm pieces
> 2 tablespoons plain flour
> 2 tablespoons (40 ml) olive oil
> 250 ml (10 fl oz) white wine
> 375 ml (15 oz) chicken stock
> 1 × 400 g (12 oz) can diced tomatoes
> 8 sprigs fresh thyme
> 1 bunch (about 500 g (20 oz) spring onions, chopped
> 3 carrots, peeled and cut into large pieces
> 600 g (24 oz) turnips, peeled and cut into large pieces
> salt and freshly ground black pepper to taste

1. Coat the pork in the flour. Heat half the oil in a large, heavy-based saucepan over a medium–high heat. Add one-quarter of the pork and cook for 3–4 minutes or until well browned. Remove from the pan and repeat with the remaining pork, adding the remaining oil when necessary. Remove all the pork from the pan.

2. Increase the heat to high and add the wine to the pan. Cook, scraping any bits off the bottom of the pan, for 2–3 minutes, or until the wine is reduced by half. Return the pork to the pan with the stock, tomatoes and thyme. Bring to the boil. Reduce the heat to low and cook, partially covered, for 30 minutes.

3. Add the spring onions, carrots and turnips to the pan. Continue to cook, partially covered, for 1 hour, or until the vegetables and meat are very tender.

Serves 6

Balsamic Lamb with Sweet Potato Mash

Per serve:	
1573 kJ/370 Cal	Protein 36 g
Fat 10.0 g	Carbohydrate 33 g
Saturated fat 3 g	GI Low

Preparation time: 10 minutes (plus 6 hours for marinating)
Cooking time: 20 minutes

> 60 ml (2 fl oz) balsamic vinegar
> 2 teaspoons (10 ml) extra-virgin olive oil
> 1 clove garlic, crushed
> 1 tablespoon fresh rosemary leaves, chopped
> 500 g (about 2 small portions) saddle of lamb (eye of loin)
> 800 g (24 oz) sweet potato, peeled, cut into chunks
> 2 tablespoons (40 ml) low fat milk*, warmed
> salt and freshly ground black pepper, to taste
> 2 teaspoons (10 ml) olive oil, extra
> 125 ml (5 fl oz) beef stock
>
> *To serve*
> 200 g (6 oz) green beans, steamed
> 400 g (12 oz) small yellow squash, steamed

1. Combine the vinegar, extra-virgin olive oil, garlic and rosemary in a shallow glass dish. Add the lamb and turn to coat. Cover and refrigerate for 6 hours or overnight to marinate.
2. Drain the lamb, reserving the marinade.
3. Cook the sweet potato until very tender. Drain well and mash until smooth. Add the milk and use a wooden spoon to beat until smooth. Season well with salt and pepper.
4. Meanwhile, heat the extra olive oil in a large frypan over a medium–high heat. Add the lamb and cook for 3–4 on minutes on each side or until cooked to your

liking. Remove the lamb from the pan and set aside. Increase the pan heat to high and add the reserved marinade and the beef stock. Simmer for 2 minutes or until the sauce reduces and thickens.

5. Divide the mash among serving plates. Thickly slice the lamb and place over the mash. Spoon the sauce over and serve with the beans and squash.

Serves 4

★ Use low fat soya milk if you prefer

Mediterranean Chicken

Per serve:	
2474 kJ/582 Cal	Protein 46 g
Fat 16.5 g	Carbohydrate 60 g
Saturated fat 3.5 g	GI Low

Preparation time: 10 minutes
Cooking time: 45 minutes

8 small chicken drumsticks
1 tablespoon (20 ml) olive oil
1 onion, peeled and cut into thin wedges
2 cloves garlic, crushed
1 × 800 g (24 oz) can diced tomatoes
175 g (7 oz) Kalamata olives
2 tablespoons tomato paste
250 g (10 oz) spirali pasta, or other short pasta
300 g (12 oz) broccoli, cut into small florets
25 g (1 oz) fresh flat leaf parsley, chopped
rind of ½ lemon, finely grated
freshly ground black pepper, to taste

1. Wrap a piece of paper towel around the end of one drumstick. Hold the paper towel with one hand and pull off the skin with the other. Discard the skin and repeat with the remaining drumsticks.
2. Heat the olive oil in a large, heavy-based saucepan over a medium heat. Add half the chicken and cook for 3–4 minutes, turning occasionally until well browned. Transfer to a plate and repeat with the remaining chicken. Set aside.
3. Add the onion and garlic to the pan and cook over a medium heat, stirring occasionally, for 4–5 minutes or until the onion softens. Return the chicken to the pan with the tomatoes, olives and tomato paste. Increase the heat and bring to the boil. Reduce the heat and

simmer, partially covered, for 20 minutes. Remove the lid and continue to cook for a further 5–10 minutes or until the chicken is cooked and the sauce thickens slightly.

4. Meanwhile, cook the pasta in a large saucepan of boiling water, following the packet directions or until *al dente*, adding the broccoli for the last minute. Drain well and return to the pan.

5. Mix the parsley and lemon rind into the pasta. Toss well to combine and season with pepper. Serve the chicken with the broccoli pasta.

Serves 4

DESSERTS AND SWEET TREATS

Fragrant Rice Pudding with Plums

As this dessert is quite high in carbs, it would be best served after a simple low carb meal such as meat or fish with salad.

Per serve:	
1258 kJ/296 Cal	Protein 10 g
Fat 4.5 g	Carbohydrate 52 g
Saturated fat 2 g	GI Low

Preparation time: 10 minutes
Cooking time: 20 minutes

100 g (4 oz) basmati rice
500 ml (20 fl oz) low fat milk
1½ tablespoons caster sugar
1 cardamom pod, lightly crushed
rind of 1 small orange, finely grated
½ teaspoon vanilla essence
½ cinnamon stick
8 plums
30 g (1 oz) pistachios, chopped, to serve

1. Cook the rice in a saucepan of boiling water for 5 minutes. Drain and return to the pan with the milk, sugar, cardamom pod, orange rind, vanilla essence and cinnamon stick.
2. Bring to the boil, then reduce the heat to low and cook, stirring regularly, for about 15–20 minutes, until the rice is tender and creamy and the liquid is almost all absorbed. Stir constantly towards the end of the cooking time, to prevent catching on the bottom.
3. Meanwhile, place the plums in a medium-sized saucepan and cover with water. Slowly bring to the

boil. Reduce the heat to very low and simmer for 10 minutes. Lift the fruit from the cooking liquid with a slotted spoon, cool slightly and slip off the skins.

4. Discard the cinnamon stick and cardamom pod from the rice, and serve immediately with the plums, sprinkled with pistachios.

Serves 4

Cherry Strudel

Per serve	
590 kJ/139 Cal	Protein 6 g
Fat 7 g	Carbohydrate 13 g
Saturated fat 2 g	GI Moderate/Medium

Preparation time: 20 minutes
Cooking time: 20 minutes

> 250 g (12 oz) reduced fat fresh ricotta
> 1 tablespoon pure floral honey
> 1 teaspoon vanilla essence
> 1 egg, lightly beaten
> 5 sheets filo pastry
> olive oil spray
> 30 g (1 oz) walnuts, finely chopped
> 250 g (12 oz) cherries, pitted

1. Preheat the oven to 190°C (375°F/gas mark 5) and line a baking tray with non-stick baking paper.
2. Place the ricotta in a bowl and mash with a fork. Add the honey, vanilla essence and egg, and mix until well combined.
3. Lay one filo sheet out on a work surface. Spray lightly with oil, and top with another sheet. Spray lightly with oil, and sprinkle evenly with walnuts. Top with the remaining pastry sheets, spraying lightly with oil (except for the last sheet).
3. Pile the ricotta mixture at one end of the pastry, and spread out leaving 3 cm bare pastry at each side and next to the end. The spread ricotta will be about 10 cm wide. Arrange the cherries over the ricotta.

4. Fold the end and sides over and roll up. Place on the prepared tray, seam side down. Spray lightly with oil and bake for 20 minutes, until golden brown. Allow to cool slightly before slicing to serve.

Serves 8

Cook's tip
Pure floral honey has a lower GI value.

Choc Nut Biscotti

Per serve	
204 kJ/48 Cal	Protein 2 g
Fat 2.5 g	Carbohydrate 5.5 g
Saturated fat 0.5 g	GI Moderate/Medium

Preparation time: 30 minutes
Cooking time: 40 minutes (plus 30 minutes' cooling time)

165 g (7 oz) caster sugar
2 eggs
160 g (6½ oz) stoneground wholemeal plain flour
60 g (2½ oz) cocoa powder
45 g (1½ oz) almonds
45 g (1½ oz) pecans
45 g (1½ oz) hazelnuts

1. Preheat the oven to 180°C (350°F/gas mark 4) and line a large baking tray with non-stick baking paper.
2. Using electric beaters, beat the sugar and eggs together for 3 minutes, until they have increased in volume, and are thick and pale.
3. Sift in the flour and cocoa powder and stir with a wooden spoon until almost combined. Add the nuts, and use clean hands to mix until well combined.
4. Divide the mixture in half and shape into 2 logs about 15 cm long. Place the logs on the tray and flatten slightly to 2 cm thick. Bake for 20 minutes, until firm. Remove from the oven and leave until completely cool.
5. Heat the oven to 120°C (250°F/gas mark 1). Cut the logs into slices about 7 mm thick. Spread out onto oven trays, and bake for 20 minutes, turning once. Cool completely on wire racks. Store in an airtight container for up to one month.

Makes about 50

Pear and Chocolate Muffins

To freeze muffins, cool them completely then wrap individually in aluminium foil. Place them in a large airtight bag, and seal. Allow to thaw at room temperature for about 1 hour.

Per serve:

863 kJ/203 Cal	Protein 5 g
Fat 6.5 g	Carbohydrate 32 g
Saturated fat 1 g	GI Moderate/Medium

Preparation time: 20 minutes
Cooking time: 20 minutes

320 g (12 oz) stoneground wholemeal flour
1 pinch of baking powder
1 teaspoon ground cinnamon
100 g (4 oz) brown sugar
1 egg
185 ml (8 fl oz) skimmed milk
2 tablespoons canola oil
2 large pears, peeled and grated
75 g (3 oz) Nutella®

1. Preheat the oven to 190°C (375°F/gas mark 5) and lightly grease a 12-cup muffin tray.
2. Sift the flour, baking powder and cinnamon into a large bowl and add in the husks. Add the sugar, combine and make a well in the centre.
3. Place the egg, milk and oil in a jug or bowl and whisk with a fork until combined. Add to the dry ingredients and fold in with a large metal spoon or rubber spatula until just combined. Do not overbeat. Gently fold in the grated pear.
4. Spoon half the mixture into the bases of each muffin recess, then place 1 teaspoon of Nutella in the centre of each. Top with the remaining mixture. Bake for 20

minutes, until risen, golden and firm to a light touch. Leave in the tins for about 3 minutes, then lift out onto a wire rack to cool.

Makes 12

Cranberry and Cinnamon Poached Pears with Custard

Per serve:

1347 kJ/317 Cal	Protein 7 g
Fat 4 g	Carbohydrate 65 g
Saturated fat 1.5 g	GI Low

Preparation time: 5 minutes
Cooking time: 40–50 minutes

> 1 litre (1¾ pints) cranberry juice
> 55 g (2 oz) caster sugar
> 3 star anise
> 1 cinnamon stick, broken
> 6 just ripe pears, peeled
>
> *Custard*
> 1 × 375 ml (15 oz) can light evaporated milk
> 2 egg yolks
> 55 g (2 oz) caster sugar
> 1 teaspoon vanilla extract

1. Place the cranberry juice, sugar, star anise and cinnamon in a medium-sized saucepan (large enough to hold the pears in a single layer). Stir over a low heat until the sugar dissolves. Increase the heat and bring to a simmer.
2. Add the pears to the poaching liquid. Cook, uncovered, for 40–50 minutes, turning occasionally until the pears are tender.
3. Meanwhile, to make the custard, heat the evaporated milk in another medium-sized saucepan until warmed through. Whisk the egg yolks, sugar and vanilla together in a heatproof bowl. Whisk the warm milk into the egg yolk mixture until well combined. Pour the mixture back into the saucepan and stir over a low heat for 10–15 minutes, or until

the custard thickens and coats the back of a wooden spoon.
4. Serve the poached pears with a little of the syrup and the custard.

Serves 6

Baked Ricotta Cheesecake

Per serve:	
1267 kJ/298 Cal	Protein 12 g
Fat 15 g	Carbohydrate 29 g
Saturated fat 6.5 g	GI Low

Preparation time: 20 minutes
Cooking time: 1 hour, 10 minutes (plus chilling time)

> ### Base
> 200 g (8 oz) packet oatmeal biscuits
> 100 g (4 oz) reduced fat margarine, melted
>
> ### Ricotta filling
> 600 g (24 oz) reduced fat fresh ricotta
> 300 g (12 oz) silken tofu, well drained
> rind of 1 lemon, finely grated
> 1 teaspoon (5 ml) vanilla extract
> 3 eggs
> 125 ml (5 oz) pure floral honey, plus extra to serve

1. Preheat the oven to 160°C (325°F/gas mark 3). Grease and line the base of a 20 cm (base measurement) springform pan with non-stick baking paper.
2. Place the biscuits in a food processor and process until fine crumbs appear. Transfer to a bowl and stir in the melted margarine. Spoon the mixture onto the base of the lined pan and use a spoon to spread evenly and press down firmly. Place in the refrigerator while you make the filling.
3. Place the ricotta, tofu, lemon rind and vanilla in a food processor and process until smooth. Add the eggs and honey and beat until smooth and well combined. Pour the ricotta mixture over the chilled base. Bake for 1 hour to 1 hour, 10 minutes or until the cheesecake is just set in the middle.
4. Turn the oven off and leave the cheesecake in the

oven with the door slightly ajar for 1 hour to cool. Set aside at room temperature until cooled completely. Cover with plastic wrap and chill for 3–4 hours.

5. To serve, drizzle each piece of cheesecake with 1 teaspoon honey.

Serves 10

Honey Oat Biscuits

Per serve:

417 kJ/98 Cal	Protein 2.5 g
Fat 5 g	Carbohydrate 11 g
Saturated fat 0.5 g	GI Moderate/Medium

Preparation time: 10 minutes
Cooking time: 25 minutes

> 125 g (5 oz) reduced fat margarine
> 125 ml (5 fl oz) pure floral honey
> 1 egg
> 75 g (3 oz) rolled oats
> 100 g (4 oz) almond meal
> 150 g (6 oz) plain flour
> ½ teaspoon ground cinnamon

1. Preheat the oven to 160°C (325°F/gas mark 3) and line two baking trays with non-stick baking paper.
2. Use electric beaters to beat the margarine and honey for 1 minute or until well combined. Add the egg and beat until combined. Stir in the oats and almond meal, then sift in the flour and cinnamon. Stir until well combined.
3. Shape tablespoons of the mixture into balls and place about 3 cm apart on the lined trays. Use a spoon to press down slightly. Bake for 10–12 minutes or until light and golden, swapping the trays around once in the oven during cooking. Transfer to a wire rack and repeat with any remaining mixture.

Makes about 24

Apple and Rhubarb Crumble

Per serve:

1300 kJ/306 Cal	Protein 7 g
Fat 13 g	Carbohydrate 33 g
Saturated fat 1.5 g	GI Low

Preparation time: 20 minutes
Cooking time: 30–40 minutes

600 g (about 3) apples (such as Golden Delicious, Pink Lady or Cox), peeled, cored and cut into quarters
1 bunch (about 670 g) rhubarb, ends trimmed, washed and cut into 4 cm lengths
2 tablespoons caster sugar

Topping
75 g (3 oz) plain flour
100 g (4 oz) almond meal
100 g (4 oz) reduced fat margarine
100 g (4 oz) untoasted muesli
firmly packed 95 g (4½ oz) brown sugar

1. Preheat the oven to 200°C (400°F/gas mark 6) and lightly grease a 2-litre ovenproof dish.
2. Layer the apples and rhubarb in the greased dish, sprinkling a little caster sugar between layers.
3. To make the crumble topping, combine the flour and almond meal in a bowl. Use your hands to rub in the margarine until well combined and large crumbs start to form. Mix in the muesli and brown sugar.
4. Sprinkle the topping evenly over the fruit. Cover the crumble with aluminium foil and bake for 20 minutes. Remove the foil and continue to cook for a further 10–20 minutes or until the fruit is tender and the crumble golden brown. Set aside for 5 minutes before serving.

Serves 8

A TO Z
GI & GL TABLES

These A to Z tables will help you put those low GI food choices into your shopping trolley and onto your plate. To make an absolutely fair comparison, all foods are tested following an internationally standardised method. Gram for gram of carbohydrate, the higher the GI, the higher the blood glucose levels after consumption.

> A **low** GI value is 55 or less
> A **moderate/medium** GI value is 56 to 69 inclusive
> A **high** GI value is 70 or more

To give you the full picture of the glycaemic impact of foods, the tables in this book also include the GL (glycaemic load) of average sized portions of the food on your plate. Glycaemic load is the product of GI and the amount of carbohydrate in a serving of food. This means that you can choose foods with either a low GI and/or a low GL.

> A **low** GL value is 10 or less
> A **moderate/medium** GL value is 11 to 19 inclusive
> A **high** GL value is 20 or more

Use the GI tables to:

- identify the best carbohydrate choices
- find the GI of your favourite foods
- compare carb-rich foods within a category (two types of bread or breakfast cereal for example)

- improve your diet by finding a low GI substitute for high GI foods

- put together a low GI meal

- help you calculate the GL of a meal or serving if it is more or less than our specified nominal portion size

Use the GL tables to:
- find foods with a high GI but low carbohydrate content per serving

Remember, the GL values listed in these tables are for the specified nominal portion size. If you eat more (or less) you will need to calculate another GL value.

We have also included some foods that contain very little carbohydrate or none at all in these tables because so many people ask us for their GI. Many vegetables such as avocado and broccoli, and protein rich foods such as eggs, cheese, chicken and tuna are among the low or no carbohydrate category. Most alcoholic beverages are also low in carbohydrate.

* indicates that this food contains little or no carbohydrate

In addition, not all low GI foods are a good choice; some are too high in saturated fat and sodium for everyday eating.

▪ indicates that this food is high in saturated fat. As we have mentioned before, the GI should not be used in isolation, but the overall nutritional value of the food needs to be considered.

If you can't find the GI value for a food you regularly eat in these tables, check out our website (www.glycemicindex.com). We maintain an international database of published GI values that have been tested by a reliable laboratory. Alternatively, contact the manufacturer and encourage them to have the food tested by a reliable laboratory. In the meantime, choose a similar food from the tables as a substitute.

Look for the GI on the foods you buy

A GI symbol on the packet tells you that a food has been glycaemic index tested. Unfortunately, not all claims are reliable.

The GI Symbol Program

This symbol on foods is your guarantee that the product meets the GI Symbol Program's strict nutritional criteria. Whether high, medium or low GI, you can be assured that these foods are healthier choices within their food group and will make a nutritious contribution to your diet.

The GI Symbol Program is an international program that was established by the University of Sydney, Diabetes Australia and the Juvenile Diabetes Research Foundation— organisations whose expertise in GI is recognised around the world. The logo is a trademark of the University of Sydney in Australia and in other countries including the UK. A food product carrying this logo is nutritious and has been tested for its GI in an accredited laboratory. For more information, visit www.gisymbol.com.

Some UK supermarket chains are progressively testing and labelling their foods. But at the time of going to press, the GI values have not been released for publication. We will include these foods in our comprehensive tables as soon as they become available and we have had an opportunity to evaluate them.

- **Sainsbury's** are launching GI labelling progressively across a range of products that meet strict nutritional

---

criteria and backing this with a comprehensive guide to GI on their website (www.sainsburys.co.uk). The products have been tested by Hammersmith Hospital Food Research Company.

- **Tesco** have had a number of foods glycaemic index tested by Oxford Brookes University and these foods are labelled low or medium GI (www.tesco.com).

Note: The GI values in this book are correct at the time of publication. However, the formulation of commercial foods can change and the GI may change as well.

Food	GI Glucose =100	Nominal serve size (g)	Available carb per serve	GL per serve
Alfalfa sprouts	*	6 g	0	0
All-Bran®, breakfast cereal, Kellogg's®	34	30 g	15	4
Angel food cake, plain	67 ■	50 g	29	19
Apple, dried	29	60 g	34	10
Apple, fresh	38	120 g	15	6
Apple juice, Granny Smith, pure	44	200 ml	24	10
Apple juice, no added sugar	40	250 ml	28	11
Apple muffin, home-made	46 ■	60 g	29	13
Apricots, canned in light syrup	64	120 g	19	12
Apricots, dried	30	60 g	28	9
Apricots, fresh	57	168 g	13	7
Arborio, risotto rice, white, boiled	69	150 g	43	29
Artichokes, globe, fresh or canned in brine	*	80 g	0	0
Arugula	*	30 g	0	0
Asparagus	*	100 g	0	0
Aubergine	*	100 g	0	0
Avocado	*	120 g	0	0
Bacon	*	50 g	0	0
Bagel, white	72	70 g	35	25
Baked beans, canned in tomato sauce	49	150 g	17	8
Banana cake, home-made	51 ■	80 g	38	18
Banana, raw	52	120 g	26	13
Banana smoothie, low fat	30	250 ml	22	7
Barley, pearled, boiled	25	150 g	32	8
Basmati rice, white, boiled	58	150 g	38	22
Bean curd, tofu, plain, unsweetened	*	100 g	0	0
Bean sprouts, raw	*	14 g	0	0
Bean thread noodles, dried, boiled	33	180 g	45	12
BEANS, PEAS & LEGUMES				
Kidney beans, dark red, canned, drained	43	150 g	25	7
Kidney beans, red, canned, drained	36	150 g	17	9
Kidney beans, red, dried, boiled	28	150 g	25	7
Beef	*	120 g	0	0
Beetroot, canned	64	80 g	7	5
Biscuits, digestive, plain	59 ■	25 g	16	10
Biscuits, Rich Tea®	55 ■	25 g	19	10
Biscuits, shortbread, plain	64 ■	25 g	16	10
Biscuits, wafer, vanilla, plain	77 ■	25 g	18	14
Black bean soup, canned	64	250 ml	27	17
Black beans, boiled	30	150 g	25	5

* little or no carbs ■ high in saturated fat

THE LOW GI GUIDE TO MANAGING PCOS

Food	GI Glucose =100	Nominal serve size (g)	Available carb per serve	GL per serve
Black rye bread	76	30 g	13	10
Black-eyed beans, soaked, boiled	42	150 g	29	12
Blueberry muffin, commercially made	59 ■	57 g	29	17
Bok choy	*	100 g	0	0
Borlotti beans, canned, drained	41	75 g	12	5
Bran Flakes™, breakfast cereal, Kellogg's®*	74	30 g	18	13
Bran muffin, commercially made	60 ■	57 g	24	15
Brawn	* ■	75 g	0	0
BREADS				
Bun, hamburger, white	61	30 g	15	9
Dark rye bread	86	30 g	14	12
Fruit loaf, thick sliced	47	30 g	15	7
Light rye bread	68	30 g	14	10
Melba toast, plain	70	30 g	23	16
Multigrain sandwich bread	65	30 g	28	18
Organic stoneground wholemeal sourdough bread	59	32 g	12	7
Pita bread, white	57	30 g	17	10
Pumpernickel bread	50	30 g	10	5
Roll (bread), white	73	30 g	16	12
Sourdough rye bread	48	30 g	12	6
Sourdough wheat bread	54	30 g	14	8
Soya and Linseed, Bürgen®	55	70 g	24	13
White bread, regular, sliced	71	30 g	14	10
BREAKFAST CEREALS				
All-Bran®, Kellogg's®	34	30 g	15	5
Bran Flakes, Kellogg's®	74	30 g	18	13
Coco Pops®, Kellogg's®	77	30 g	26	20
Corn Flakes®, Kellogg's®	77	30 g	25	20
Crunchy Nut Corn Flakes Bar, Kellogg's®	72	30 g	26	19
Crunchy Nut Corn Flakes, breakfast cereal, Kellogg's®	72	30 g	24	17
Frosties®, Kellogg's®	55	30 g	26	15
Oat bran, raw, unprocessed	55	10 g	5	3
Oats, rolled, raw	59	50 g	31	18
BREAKFAST CEREALS				
Porridge, instant, made with water	82	30 g	26	17
Porridge, regular, made from oats with water	58	250 g	21	11
Puffed Wheat	80	30 g	21	17
Rice Krispies®, Kellogg's®	82	30 g	26	22
Semolina, cooked	55	150 g	11	6

* little or no carbs ■ high in saturated fat

Food	GI Glucose =100	Nominal serve size (g)	Available carb per serve	GL per serve
BREAKFAST CEREALS (continued)				
Shredded Wheat	75	30 g	20	15
Special K®, regular, Kellogg's®	56	30 g	21	11
Sultana Bran™, Kellogg's®	73	30 g	19	14
Broad beans	79	80 g	11	9
Broccoli	*	60 g	0	0
Brussels sprouts	*	100 g	0	0
Buckwheat, boiled	54	150 g	30	16
Buckwheat, puffed	65	14 g	12	8
Bulghur, cracked wheat, ready to eat	48	150 g	26	12
Bun, hamburger, white	61	30 g	15	9
Butter beans, canned, drained	36	75 g	12	4
Butter beans, dried, boiled	31	150 g	20	6
Cabbage	*	70 g	0	0
Cake, chocolate, made from packet mix with icing	38■	111 g	52	20
Cake, cupcake, strawberry-iced	73■	38 g	26	19
Cake, pound, plain	54■	50 g	23	12
Cake, sponge, plain, unfilled	46■	63 g	36	17
Calamari rings, squid, not battered or crumbed	*	70 g	0	0
Cannellini beans	31	85 g	12	4
Cantaloupe	67	120 g	6	4
Carrot juice, freshly made	43	250 ml	23	10
Carrots, peeled, boiled	41	80 g	5	2
Cashew nuts, salted	22	30 g	9	2
Cauliflower	*	60 g	0	0
Celery	*	40 g	0	0
CEREAL GRAINS				
Rye, grain	34	50 g	38	13
Cheese	*■	120 g	0	0
Cheese tortellini, cooked	50■	180 g	21	10
Cherries, dark, raw	63	120 g	12	3
Chicken	*	110 g	0	0
Chicken nuggets, frozen, reheated in microwave 5 mins	46■	100 g	16	7
Chickpeas, canned in brine	40	150 g	22	9
Chickpeas, dried, boiled	28	150 g	24	7
Chillies, fresh or dried	*	20 g	0	0
Chives, fresh	*	4 g	0	0
Chocolate cake, made from packet mix with icing	38■	110 g	52	20
Chocolate, dark, plain	41■	30 g	19	8
Chocolate, milk, plain, Cadbury's®	49■	30 g	17	8

* little or no carbs ■ high in saturated fat

THE LOW GI GUIDE TO MANAGING PCOS

Food	GI Glucose =100	Nominal serve size (g)	Available carb per serve	GL per serve
Chocolate, white, plain, Nestlé®	44 ■	50 g	29	13
Coca-Cola®, soft drink	53	250 ml	26	14
Coco Pops®, breakfast cereal, Kellogg's®	77	30 g	26	20
Condensed milk, sweetened, full fat	61 ■	50 ml	28	17
Consommé, clear, chicken or vegetable	*	205 g	2	0
Corn, sweet, on the cob, boiled	48	80 g	16	8
Corn, sweet, whole kernel, canned, drained	46	80 g	14	7
Cornflakes, breakfast cereal, Kellogg's®	77	30 g	25	20
Cornmeal (polenta), boiled	68	150 g	13	9
Courgette	*	100 g	0	0
Couscous, boiled 5 mins	65	150 g	33	21
Cranberries, dried, sweetened	64	40 g	29	19
Cranberry Juice Cocktail, Ocean Spray	52	250 ml	31	16
Croissant, plain	67 ■	57 g	26	17
Crumpet, white	69	50 g	19	13
Crunchy Nut Corn Flakes Bar, Kellogg's®	72	30 g	26	19
Crunchy Nut Corn Flakes Bar, Kellogg's®	72	30 g	26	19
Cucumber	*	45 g	0	0
Cupcake, strawberry-iced	73 ■	38 g	26	19
Custard apple, fresh, flesh only	54	120 g	19	10
Custard, home-made from milk, wheat starch and sugar	43 ■	100 ml	17	7
Custard, vanilla, reduced fat	37	100 ml	15	6
Dark rye bread	86	30 g	14	12
Dates, Arabic, dried, vacuum-packed	39	55 g	41	16
Dates, dried	103	60 g	40	42
Desiree potato, peeled, boiled 35 mins	101	150 g	17	17
Diet jelly, made from crystals with water	*	125 g	0	0
Diet soft drinks	*	250 ml	0	0
Digestive biscuits, plain	59 ■	25 g	16	10
Dried apple	29	60 g	34	10
Duck	* ■	140 g	0	0
Eggs	* ■	120 g	0	0
Endive	*	30 g	0	0
Fanta®, orange soft drink	68	250 ml	34	23

* little or no carbs ■ high in saturated fat

Food	GI Glucose =100	Nominal serve size (g)	Available carb per serve	GL per serve
Fat-free yoghurts, various flavours	40	200 g	31	12
Fennel	*	90 g	0	0
Fettuccine, egg, cooked	40	180 g	46	18
Figs, dried, tenderised	61	60 g	26	16
Fish	*	120 g	0	0
Fish fingers	38■	100 g	19	7
Four bean mix, canned, drained	37	75 g	12	5
French fries, frozen, reheated in microwave	75■	150 g	29	22
Frosties®, breakfast cereal, Kellogg's®	55	30 g	26	15
Fructose, pure	19	10 g	10	2
Fruit loaf, thick sliced	54	30 g	15	8
Garlic	*	5 g	0	0
Ginger	*	10 g	0	0
Glucose tablets	100	10 g	10	10
Glutinous rice, white, cooked in rice cooker	98	150 g	32	31
Gnocchi, cooked	68	180 g	48	33
Golden syrup	63	20 g	17	11
Granny Smith apple juice, unsweetened	44	200 ml	24	10
Grapefruit, fresh	25	120 g	11	3
Grapefruit juice, unsweetened	48	250 ml	22	9
Grapes, fresh	53	120 g	18	8
Green beans	*	70 g	0	0
Green pea soup, canned	66	250 ml	41	27
Ham, leg or shoulder	*■	24 g	0	0
Hamburger bun, white	61	30 g	15	9
Haricot beans, cooked, canned	38	150 g	31	12
Haricot beans, dried, boiled	33	150 g	31	12
Heinz® Baked Beans in tomato sauce, canned	49	150 g	17	8
Herbs, fresh or dried	*	2 g	0	0
Hommous, regular	6	30 g	5	1
Honey and Oat Bran Bread, Vogel's	49	40 g	13	7
Honey, pure floral	35	25 g	18	6
Honey, various (averaged)	55	25 g	18	10
Ice-cream, vanilla, full fat	38■	50 g	9	3
Instant mashed potato	85	150 g	20	17
Instant noodles, 99% fat free	67	75 g	51	34
Instant noodles, regular	54■	180 g	23	10
Instant rice, white, cooked 6 mins	87	150 g	42	36
Isostar® sports drink	70	250 ml	18	13

* little or no carbs ■ high in saturated fat   197

Food	GI Glucose =100	Nominal serve size (g)	Available carb per serve	GL per serve
Jasmine rice, white, long-grain, cooked in rice cooker	109	150 g	42	46
Jelly beans	78	30 g	28	22
Jelly, diet, made from crystals with water	*	125 g	0	0
Kidney beans, dark red, canned, drained	43	150 g	25	7
Kidney beans, red, canned, drained	36	150 g	17	9
Kidney beans, red, dried, boiled	28	150 g	25	7
Kiwi fruit, fresh	53	120 g	12	6
Lamb	*	120 g	0	0
Leeks	*	80 g	0	0
Lemon	*	40 g	0	0
Lentil soup, canned	44	250 ml	21	9
Lentils, green, dried, boiled	30	150 g	17	5
Lentils, red, dried, boiled	26	150 g	18	5
Lettuce	*	50 g	0	0
Licorice, soft	78	60 g	42	33
Light rye bread	68	30 g	14	10
Lima beans, baby, frozen, reheated in microwave	32	150 g	30	10
Lime	*	40 g	0	0
Linguine pasta, thick, durum wheat, boiled	46	180 g	48	22
Linguine pasta, thin, durum wheat, boiled	52	180 g	45	23
Linseed and Soya Loaf, bread	55	70 g	24	13
Liver sausage	*■	30 g	0	0
Low-fat soya milk, calcium-fortified	44	250 ml	17	8
Lucozade®, original, sparkling glucose drink	95	250 ml	42	40
Lychees, canned, in syrup, drained	79	120 g	20	16
M&M's®, peanut	33■	30 g	17	6
Macaroni, white, plain, boiled	47	180 g	48	23
Mango, fresh	51	120 g	17	8
Maple syrup, pure, Canadian	54	24 g	18	10
Mars Bar®, regular	62■	60 g	40	25
Marshmallows, plain, pink and white	62	25 g	20	12
Melba toast, plain	70	30 g	23	16
Milk, semi-skimmed, low fat (1.4%)	32	250 ml	12	4
Milk, skimmed, low fat (0.1%)	32	250 ml	12	4
Milk, soya, calcium-enriched	36	250 ml	18	6
Milk, soya, calcium-enriched	36	250 ml	18	6

∗ little or no carbs ■ high in saturated fat

Food	GI Glucose =100	Nominal serve size (g)	Available carb per serve	GL per serve
Milky Bar®, plain white chocolate, Nestlé®	44 ■	50 g	29	13
Minestrone soup, traditional, canned	39	250 g	18	7
Muesli bar, chewy, with choc chips or fruit	54 ■	31 g	21	12
Muesli bar, crunchy, with dried fruit	61	30 g	21	13
Muffins, apple, home-made	46 ■	60 g	29	13
Muffins, blueberry, commercially made	59 ■	57 g	29	17
Muffins, bran, commercially made	60 ■	57 g	24	15
Multigrain sandwich bread	65	30 g	28	18
Mung bean noodles (bean thread), dried, boiled	33	180 g	45	18
Mung beans	39	150 g	17	5
Mushrooms	*	35 g	0	0
New potato, canned, microwaved 3 mins	65	150 g	18	12
New potato, unpeeled and boiled 20 mins	78	150 g	21	13
Noodles 2 minute, regular, Maggi	54	75 g	51	34
Noodles 2 minute, (99% fat free), Maggi	71	75 g	51	34
Nutella®, hazelnut spread	33	20 g	12	4
Nuts, peanuts, roasted, salted	14	50 g	6	1
Nuts, pecan, raw	10	50 g	3	1
Oat bran, unprocessed	55	10 g	5	3
Oatcakes	57 ■	25 g	15	8
Oats, rolled, raw	59	50 g	31	18
Okra	*	80 g	0	0
Onions, raw, peeled	*	30 g	0	0
Orange, fresh	42	120 g	11	5
Orange juice, unsweetened	50	250 ml	18	9
Organic stoneground wholemeal sourdough bread	59	32 g	12	7
Oysters, natural, plain	*	85 g	0	0
Parsnips	97	80 g	12	12
PASTA				
Cheese tortellini, cooked	50 ■	180 g	21	10
Fettuccine, egg, cooked	40	180 g	46	18
Gnocchi, cooked	68	180 g	48	33
Linguine, thick, durum wheat, boiled	46	180 g	48	22
Linguine, thin, durum wheat, boiled	52	180 g	45	23
Macaroni, white, plain, boiled	47	180 g	48	23

N

O

P

THE LOW GI GUIDE TO MANAGING PCOS

Food	GI Glucose =100	Nominal serve size (g)	Available carb per serve	GL per serve
PASTA (continued)				
Ravioli, meat-filled, durum wheat flour, boiled	39 ■	180 g	38	15
Rice pasta, brown, boiled	92	180 g	38	35
Spaghetti, white, durum wheat, boiled 10–15 mins	44	180 g	48	21
Spaghetti, wholemeal, boiled	42	180 g	42	16
Spirali, white, durum wheat, boiled	43	180 g	44	19
Vermicelli, white, durum wheat, boiled	35	180 g	44	16
Paw paw, fresh	56	120 g	8	5
Peach, fresh	42	120 g	11	5
Peaches, canned, in heavy syrup	58	120 g	15	9
Peaches, canned, in light syrup	57	120 g	18	9
Peaches, canned, in natural juice	45	120 g	11	4
Peanuts, roasted, salted	14	50 g	6	1
Pear, fresh	38	120 g	11	4
Pear halves, canned, in natural juice	44	120 g	13	5
Pear halves, canned, in reduced-sugar syrup	25	120 g	14	4
Peas, dried, boiled	22	150 g	9	2
Peas, green, frozen, boiled	48	80 g	7	3
Pecan nuts, raw	10	50 g	3	1
Pineapple, fresh	59	120 g	10	6
Pineapple juice, unsweetened	46	250 ml	34	16
Pita bread, white	57	30 g	17	10
Pizza, Super Supreme, pan, Pizza Hut	36 ■	100 g	24	9
Pizza, Super Supreme, thin and crispy, Pizza Hut *	30 ■	100 g	22	7
Plum, raw	39	120 g	12	5
Polenta, boiled	68	150 g	13	9
Polos®	70	30 g	30	21
Pop-Tarts™, choctastic	70	50 g	36	25
Popcorn, plain, cooked in microwave	72	20 g	11	8
Pork	* ■	120 g	0	0
Porridge, instant, made with water	82	30 g	26	17
Porridge, regular, made from oats with water	58	250 g	21	11
Potato crisps, plain, salted	54 ■	50 g	18	10
POTATOES				
Desiree, peeled, boiled 35 mins	101	150 g	17	17
French fries, frozen, reheated in microwave	75 ■	150 g	29	22
Instant mashed potato	85	150 g	20	17

Food	GI Glucose =100	Nominal serve size (g)	Available carb per serve	GL per serve
POTATOES (continued)				
New, canned, microwaved 3 mins	65	150 g	18	12
New, unpeeled, boiled 20 mins	78	150 g	21	13
Sweet potato, baked	46	150 g	25	11
Pound cake, plain	54 ■	50 g	23	12
Pretzels, oven-baked, traditional wheat flavour	83	30 g	20	16
Prunes, pitted	29	60 g	33	10
Puffed rice cakes, white	82	25 g	21	17
Puffed Wheat, breakfast cereal	80	30 g	21	17
Pumpernickel bread	50	30 g	10	5
Pumpkin	75	80 g	4	3
Quinoa, organic, boiled	53	100 g	17	9
Radishes	*	15 g	0	0
Raisins	64	60 g	44	28
Raspberries	*	65 g	0	0
Ravioli, meat-filled, durum wheat flour, boiled	39 ■	180 g	38	15
Rhubarb	*	125 g	0	0
Rice cakes, puffed, white	82	25 g	21	17
Rice noodles, dried, boiled	61	176 g	39	24
Rice noodles, fresh, boiled	40	180 g	39	15
Rice pasta, brown, gluten-free, boiled	92	180 g	38	35
Rice vermicelli, dried, boiled	58	180 g	39	22
Risotto rice, Arborio, boiled	69	150 g	43	29
Rockmelon	65	12 g	6	4
Roll (bread), white	73	30 g	16	12
Rye bread, wholemeal	51	40 g	13	7
Rye, grain	34	50 g	38	13
Ryvita® crispbread*	69	25 g	16	11
Salami	* ■	120 g	0	0
Salmon, fresh or canned in water or brine	*	150 g	0	0
Sardines	*	60 g	0	0
Sausages, fried	28 ■	100 g	3	1
Scallops, natural, plain	*	160 g	0	0
Scones, plain, made from packet mix	92	25 g	9	8
Semolina, cooked	55	150 g	11	6
Shallots	*	10 g	0	0
Shredded Wheat breakfast cereal	75	30 g	20	15
Skimmed milk, low fat (0.1%)	32	250 ml	12	4
Skittles®	70 ■	50 g	45	32
Sourdough bread, organic, stoneground, wholemeal	59	32 g	12	7

* little or no carbs ■ high in saturated fat

Food	GI Glucose =100	Nominal serve size (g)	Available carb per serve	GL per serve
Sourdough rye bread	48	30 g	12	6
Sourdough wheat bread	54	30 g	14	8
Soya and Linseed, Bürgen®	55	70 g	24	13
Soya milk, calcium-enriched	36	250 ml	18	6
Soya milk, low-fat, calcium-fortified	44	250 ml	17	8
Soya yoghurt, Peach and Mango, 2% fat	50	200 g	26	13
Soyabeans, canned	14	150 g	6	1
Soyabeans, dried, boiled	18	150 g	6	1
Spaghetti, gluten-free, rice and split pea, canned in tomato sauce	68	220 g	27	19
Spaghetti, white, durum wheat, boiled 10–15 mins	44	180 g	48	21
Spaghetti, wholemeal, boiled	42	180 g	42	16
Special K®, regular, breakfast cereal, Kellogg's®	56	30 g	21	11
Spinach	*	75 g	0	0
Spirali pasta, white, durum wheat, boiled	43	180 g	44	19
Split pea soup, canned	60	250 ml	27	16
Sponge cake, plain, unfilled	46 ■	63 g	36	17
Spring onions	*	15 g	0	0
Squash, yellow	*	70 g	0	0
Squid or calamari, not battered or crumbed	*	70 g	0	0
Steak, any cut	* ■	120 g	0	0
Strawberries, fresh	40	120 g	3	1
Strawberry jam, regular	51	30 g	20	10
Sugar	68	10 g	10	7
Sultana Bran™, breakfast cereal, Kellogg's®	73	30 g	19	14
Sultanas	56	60 g	45	25
Sushi, salmon	48	100 g	36	17
Swede, cooked	72	150 g	10	7
Sweet corn, on the cob, boiled	48	80 g	16	8
Sweet corn, whole kernel, canned, drained	46	80 g	14	7
Sweet potato, baked	46	150 g	25	11
Sweetened condensed full fat milk	61 ■	50 g	28	17
Sweetened dried cranberries	64	40 g	29	19
Taco shells, cornmeal-based, baked	68	20 g	12	8
Taro	54	150 g	8	4
Tofu (bean curd), plain, unsweetened	*	100 g	0	0
Tomato	*	150 g	0	0

* little or no carbs ■ high in saturated fat

Food	GI Glucose =100	Nominal serve size (g)	Available carb per serve	GL per serve
Tomato juice, no added sugar	38	250 ml	9	4
Tomato soup, canned	45	250 ml	17	6
Tortellini, cheese, boiled	50■	180 g	21	10
Trout, fresh or frozen	*	63 g	0	0
Tuna, fresh or canned in water or brine	*	120 g	0	0
Turkey	*■	140 g	0	0
Twix® bar	44■	60 g	39	17
Vanilla cake made from packet mix with vanilla frosting,	42■	111 g	58	24
Vanilla custard, reduced fat	37	100 g	15	6
Vanilla ice-cream, full fat	38■	50 g	9	3
Veal	*	120 g	0	0
Vermicelli, white, durum wheat, boiled	35	180 g	44	16
Vinegar	*	5 ml	0	0
Vogel's honey and oat bran bread	49	40 g	13	7
Wafer biscuits, vanilla, plain	77■	25 g	18	14
Water crackers, plain	78	25 g	18	14
Watercress	*	8 g	0	0
Watermelon, raw	76	120 g	6	4
Wheat, cracked, bulghur, ready to eat	48	150 g	26	12
White bread, regular, sliced	71	30 g	14	10
Wholemeal rye bread	51	40g	13	7
Wild rice, boiled	57	164 g	32	18
Yam, peeled, boiled	37	150 g	36	13
Yoghurt, diet, low fat, no added sugar, vanilla or fruit (averaged)	20	200 g	13	3
Yoghurt, Ski™, low fat, with sugar, Strawberry	33	200 g	31	10

V

W

Y

Note

The GI of the brand-name items listed in the tables has been derived from *in vivo* testing by reliable laboratories in various countries around the world. Because processing procedures may vary from country to country, products manufactured in the UK may or may not have identical values.

* little or no carbs ■ high in saturated fat

GLOSSARY

Acanthosis nigricans: sandpaper-like dark skin located in the skin of armpits, root of the neck and, in severe cases, over joints. It is the result of severe insulin resistance. Not uncommonly, patients describe it as 'dirty skin' that cannot be washed off !

Amenorrhea: when a woman has had no periods in her lifetime.

Anabolic hormone: any steroid, including synthetic preparations, which enhances constructive metabolism. They are notorious for their abuse by athletes to increase the size of their muscles.

Androstenedione: a male sex hormone weaker in activity than testosterone, produced by the ovary, testis and adrenal glands. The body can convert it to both male and female sex-steroids.

Corpus luteum: a group of cells associated with bringing the egg to maturity. It secretes the hormone progesterone in anticipation of pregnancy.

Dianette: (also known as Diane) a pill used widely as a combination contraceptive and a means of controlling acne and hirsutism. One of its two components, cyproterone acetate, suppresses ovarian function (and in large doses, over a long period of time, also adrenal function). The second component, a synthetic estrogen, puts back the estrogen into the body.

Dyslipidaemia: abnormal levels or composition of blood fats. Because these fats are water insoluble they are ferried around on proteins. These ferrying proteins specialise in the load they carry and differ in size depending on how much fat they are carrying. The 'good cholesterol' is carried on a very distinct protein from the one that carries the 'bad cholesterol' and those that carry triglycerides, a complex of fatty acid absorbed from food.

Fatty liver: is the build up of excessive amounts of triglycerides and other fats inside liver cells; also known as Steatohepatitis or NASH.

Follicle-stimulating hormone (FSH): a hormone produced by the pituitary gland. It affects women's ovaries, stimulating the production of an egg cell.

Glycaemic load: a measure of the glycaemic impact of foods based on both the type and amount of carbohydrate. It is calculated by multiplying the GI of a food by the available carbohydrate content (carbohydrate minus fibre) in a serving (expressed in grams), divided by 100.

Glycaemic potential: the predicted blood glucose raising effect that a food contains.

Hirsutism: excessive growth of hair of normal or abnormal distribution. Excessive body-hair growth may be interpreted differently depending on ethnicity, complexion and hair colour. For example, relatively heavy dark body-hair growth is the rule in dark women of Mediterranean origin but may be abnormal in a blonde Swede, particularly if thick and wiry. This type of hair growth on the face, around the nipples, between the breasts, lower back, up the naval line and inside the thighs is decidedly worthy of attention.

Hypoglycemia: a condition that occurs when one's blood glucose is lower than normal, usually less than 4 mmol/L. Signs include hunger, nervousness, shakiness, perspiration, dizziness or light-headedness, sleepiness and confusion. If left untreated, hypoglycemia may lead to unconciousness.

Hypothalamus: a basal part of the central region of the brain that contains many regulatory centres including ones that send periodic signals to the pituitary gland, which in turn secretes specific hormones. Contrary to previous belief that the pituitary was 'the master gland', with better knowledge, much of that role appears to lie with the hypothalamus.

Insulin resistance: if you are insulin resistant, your muscle and liver cells are not good at taking up glucose unless there's a lot of insulin about. Chances are you'll have very high insulin levels even long after a meal, as your body tries hard to metabolise the carbohydrate in the meal.

Luteinising hormone (LH): a hormone produced by the pituitary gland. It plays a role in the initial production of egg cells by the ovary.

Menarche: stage of sexual development in a girl marked by the first period.

Pituitary gland: a small oval endocrine organ connected by a stalk to the hypothalamus. It is made up of two parts: the anterior (that facing forward) is involved in making and secreting several hormones including FSH and LH.

Pre-eclampsia: a serious complication of late pregnancy characterised by a sudden increase in blood pressure, excessive weight gain, swelling and protein in the urine. It requires immediate medical attention.

Sex hormones: a generic term to cover male and female sex hormones produced by testis, ovary and adrenal gland.

USEFUL CONTACTS

Useful websites:
http://www.verity-pcos.org.uk

The main resource for women with PCOS in the UK.

http://www.diagnosemefirst.com

A comprehensive website covering many of the aspects of PCOS and linked conditions.

http://www.hairfacts.com

Hair removal products tried and tested. Also links to buy products online.

http://www.bda.uk.com

A good place to start looking for a dietitian near you.

http://www.pcosupport.org

A US-based website with information on PCOS and a noticeboard where reader queries are addressed by other readers.

http://www.glycemicindex.com

A searchable GI database that is updated regularly.

http://www.whi.org.uk

This community based website provides plenty of programmes based activity on walking and steps.

REFERENCES

E. Carmina & R. A. Lobo, 'Polycystic ovary syndrome (PCOS): arguably the most common endocrinopathy is associated with significant morbidity in women.' *Journal of Clinical Endocrinology and Metabolism* 84, 1999, pp. 1897–1899.

A. Garg & A. Misra, 'Hepatic steatosis, insulin resistance and adipose tissue disorders.' *Journal of Clinical Endocrinology and Metabolism* 87, 2002, pp. 3019–3022.

A. Dunaif, 'Insulin resistance and the polycystic ovarian syndrome: Mechanisms and implications for pathogenesis.' *Endocrine Reviews* 18, 1997, pp. 774–800.

R. Kaaja, H. Laivuori, M. Laasko, M.J. Tikkanen, and O. Ylikorakala, 'Evidence of a state of increased insulin resistance in pre-eclampsia.' *Metabolism* 48, 1999, pp. 892–896.

A.N. Vgontzas, R.S. Legro, A. Bixler, A. Grayerv, A. Kales and G.P. Chrousos, 'Polycystic ovarian syndrome is associated with obstructive sleep apnoea and daytime sleepiness: Role of insulin resistance.' *Journal of Clinical Endocrinology and Metabolism* 86, 2001, pp. 517–520.

V.L. Nelson, K.N. Qin, R.L. Rosenfield, J.R. Wood, T.M. Penning, R.S. Legro, J.F. Straus II and J.M. McAllister, 'The biochemical basis for increased testosterone production in theca cells propagated from patients with polycystic ovarian disease.' *Journal of Clinical Endocrinology and Metabolism* 86, 2001, pp. 5925–5923.

A.M. Corbould, S.J. Judd and R.J. Rodger's, 'Expression of types 1, 2, 3 and 3 17 beta-hyroxesteroid dehydrogenase in subcutaneous abdominal and intra-abdominal adipose tissue of women.' *Journal of Clinical Endocrinology and Metabolism* 83, 2001, pp. 187–194.

B.O. Yildiz, H. Yarali, H. Oguz and M. Bayraktar, 'Glucose intolerance, insulin resistance, and hyperandrogenemia in first degree relatives of women with polycystic ovary syndrome.' *Journal of Clinical Endocrinology and Metabolism* 88, 2003, pp. 2031–2036.

M. Urbanek, R.S. Legro, D.A. Driscoll, R. Azziz, D.A. Ehrmann, R.J. Norman, J.F. Strauss 3rd, R.S. Spielman and A.Dunaif, 'Thirty-seven candidate genes for polycystic ovary syndrome: Strongest evidence for linkage is with follistatin.' *Proceedings of the National Academy of Science of the United States of America* 96, 1999, pp. 8573–8.

D.J. Jakubowicz, M.J. Iuorno, S. Jakubowicz, K.A. Roberts and J.E Nestler, 'Effects of metformin on early pregnancy loss in polycystic ovary syndrome.' *Journal of Clinical Endocrinology and Metabolism* 87, 2001, pp. 524–529.

N.L. Ragon, R.C. Rao, S. Hwang, L.L. Alshuter, S. Elman, L. Zuckerbrow-Miller and S.G. Korenman, 'Depression in women with polycystic ovarian disease: Clinical and biochemical correlates' *Journal of Affective Disorders* 3, 2003, pp. 299–304.

D. Kirpichnikov, S.I. McFarklane, J.R. Sowers, 'Metformin: An update.' *Annals of Internal Medicine*, 2002, pp. 25-33.

A. Azziz, 'The evaluation and management of hirsutism.' *Obstetrics and Gynecology* 101, 2003, pp.995–1007.

R. E. Frisch, *Female Fertility and the Body Fat Connection*, University of Chicago Press, London, 2002.

S. B. Zweig, M.C.Tolentino and L. Portesky, 'Polycystic ovarian disease' in *Principles of Diabetes Mellitus* L. Poretsky (ed.) Kluwer Academic Publishers, Boston, 2002, pp. 701–721.

J. Diamond, 'The double puzzle of diabetes' *Nature* 423, 2002, pp. 599–602.

J.C. Brand-Miller and S. Colagiuri, 'The carnivore connection: dietary carbohydrate in the evolution of NIDDM.' *Diabetologia* 37, 1994, pp. 1280–1286.

G.Taubes, 'Insulin insults may spur Alzheimer's disease.' *Science* 301, 2003, pp. 40–41.

J.M. Lord, I.H. Flight & R.J. Norman, 'Metformin in polycystic ovary disease syndrome: systematic review and metanalysis.' *British Medical Journal* 327, 2003, pp. 951–953.

D.J. Jakubowicz, P.A. Essah, M. Seppala, S. Jakubowics, J.P. Baillargeon, R. Koistinen, & J.F. Nestler, 'Reduced serum glycodelin and insulin-like growth factor protein-1 in women with polycystic ovarian syndrome during the first trimester of pregnancy.' *Journal of Clinical Endocrinology and Metabolism* 89, 2004, pp. 933–839.

C.J. Glueck, N. Goldenberg, J. Pranikoff, M. Loftspring, L. Sieve & P. Wang, 'Height, weight and motor-social development during the first 18 months of life in 126 infants born to 109 mothers with polycystic ovary syndrome who conceived and continued through pregnancy.' *Human Reproduction* 19, 2004, pp. 1323–1330.

L. Ibanez, C. Valla, S. Cabre & F. de Zegher, 'Flutamide-metformin plus ethinylestradiol-drospirenone for lipolysis and antiatherogenesis in young women with ovarian hyperandrogenism: the key role of early, low-dose flutamide.' *Journal of Clinical Endocrinology and Metabolism* 89, 2004, pp. 4716–4720.

L. Ibanez, C. Valls, N. Ptau, M.V. Marcus & F. de Zegher, 'Polycystic ovary syndrome after precocious pubarche: ontogeny of low-birthweight effect.' *Clinical Endocrinology* 55, 2001, pp. 667–672.

E. Diamanti-Kandararakis, C. Houli, K. Alexandraki & G. Spina, 'Failure of mathematical indices to accurately assess insulin resistance in lean, overweight, or obese women with polycystic ovary syndrome.' *Journal of Clinical Endocrinology and Metabolism* 89, 2004, pp. 1273–1276.

C. Holden, 'Long-term stress may chip away at the ends of chromosomes.' *Science* 306, 2004, p. 1666.

U. Özcan, Q. Cao, E. Yilmax, A-H. Lee, N.N. Iwakoshi, E. Özleden, G. Tuncman, C. Görgün, L.H. Glimcher & G.S Hotamisligil, 'Endoplasmic reticulum stress links obesity, insulin action, and type 2 diabetes.' *Science* 306, 2004, pp. 457–461.

Professor Jennie Brand-Miller holds a Personal Chair in Human Nutrition in the School of Molecular and Microbial Biosciences at the University of Sydney in Sydney, Australia. In 2003 she was awarded a Clunies Ross National Science and Technology Medal for her work in championing a new approach to nutrition and the management of blood glucose. Her research interests have focused on all aspects of carbohydrates—diet and diabetes, the glycaemic index of foods, insulin resistance, lactose intolerance and oligosaccharides in infant nutrition. She holds a special interest in evolutionary nutrition and the diet of Australian Aborigines. She has published seventeen books and over 200 peer-reviewed journal articles. *The New Glucose Revolution*, the worldwide bestselling series on the glycaemic index, co-authored by Kaye Foster-Powell and Stephen Colagiuri, has been translated into 14 languages.

Professor Nadir R. Farid began his academic career at the Memorial University of Newfoundland, Canada. He became Professor of Medicine and Endocrinology in 1984 and of Cell Sciences in 1989. He is an internationally recognised investigative and clinical endocrinologist who has trained many scientists, internists and endocrinologists, and described or redefined a number of clinical syndromes. His specialist interests are the genetics of endocrine disorders and the molecular basis of thyroid cancer. He has edited five books and published in excess of 450 scientific papers, reviews and chapters. He is founder and CEO of Osancor Biotech Inc and consultant at 119 Harley Street and The Wellington Hospital, both in London.

Kate Marsh

Kate Marsh is an Accredited Practising Dietitian and Diabetes Educator, with a Masters of Nutrition and Dietetics from the University of Sydney (1995) and a Graduate Certificate in Diabetes Education and Management from the University of Technology, Sydney (1997). She has worked in private practice in Australia for eight years, combining this for the first three years with her position as dietitian and diabetes educator at Hornsby Ku-ring-gai Hospital, and now works full time in private practice. Kate has a particular interest in PCOS, having worked with hundreds of women with this condition over the past few years. She is currently undertaking her PhD at the University of Sydney looking at the benefits of a low GI diet in the management of insulin resistance in women with PCOS.

INDEX

INDEX

RECIPE INDEX

**Transform your life
with Hodder Mobius**

For the latest information on the best in
Spirituality, Self Help,
Health & Wellbeing and Parenting,

visit our website
www.hoddermobius.com

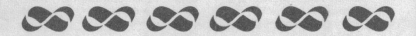

Other books in the Low GI series

The Low GI Diet
The Low GI Life Plan
The Low GI Guide to the Metabolic Syndrome and your Heart
The Low GI Shopper's Guide to GI Values
Low GI Eating Made Easy
The New Glucose Revolution
The Glucose Revolution & Children with Type 1 Diabetes
The Glucose Revolution & Healthy Children
The Glucose Revolution & Losing Weight
The Glucose Revolution & Sports Nutrition
The Glucose Revolution for People with Diabetes